LICHEN SCLEROSUS

BODY, MIND & SPIRIT PRACTICES TO HEAL THE STRESS OF LS

STEPHANIE HREHIRCHUK

StephanieHrehirchuk.com

Lichen Sclerosus: Body, Mind & Spirit Practices to Heal the Stress of LS

by Stephanie Hrehirchuk

Editor: Maraya Loza Koxahn

Cover image: Canva

Cover design: Stephanie Hrehirchuk

Interior design: Stephanie Hrehirchuk

ISBN print 978-1-9991300-9-1

ISBN ebook 978-1-7782301-0-3

CONTENTS

DISCLAIMER

The information presented here represents the view of the author as of the date of publication. This book is meant to inform, not diagnose or treat specific health conditions. It is not a substitute for professional medical advice, diagnosis and treatment. Always consult your doctor or health care practitioner.

This book is dedicated to the entire LS community

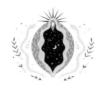

INTRODUCTION

"There's no way every woman in menopause feels this pain." I tried to get my point across to my doctor without becoming a difficult patient. "Having sex feels like broken glass!"

Looking back, I wish I *had* been a more difficult patient. I'd accepted the pat on the head and the menopause diagnosis and then continued to watch my vulva, along with my sex life and marriage, disappear. That was four years ago.

I turned 50 last November and decided that was my year to make my doctor listen. I booked my pap, informed my doctor of all the pain and discomfort I'd experienced over the years and then awaited the results. My doctor called the following week with the all-clear. *That can't be.* I pulled out a mirror and did my own inspection; something I should have done much sooner but was occupied with the perfect storm of divorce, single parenting, selling the family home, and Covid. I did not agree with her opinion. I also did not know the difference between vulva and vagina, part of the great education I've received while digging into the details of menopause health.

From The Menopause Centre (Vulva-Vaginal Disorders Specialist & Vulva Dermatology):

The vulva includes the mons (the hairy area), the labia majora (large lips, also hairy), the labia minora (small lips that you can see when you spread the large lips, the clitoris and clitoral hood (the hood partially covers the top of the clitoris), the urethra (where the urine comes out), the vaginal opening, the perineum (behind the vagina and in front of the anus. and the perianal area (Area around the anus).[1]

Yourdictionary.com defines the vagina as:

The definition of a **vagina** is the passage leading from the vulva to the cervix...[2]

It didn't take long for Google to diagnose the issue. The more I read, the angrier and sadder I became. Sad-mad. Now, I don't typically recommend using Dr. Google as your healthcare practitioner, however, I'd already told my doctor about the pain and that I'd received no relief in years. I needed to get to the bottom of this misdiagnosed issue.

I called the doctor's office the next day and booked a phone consultation. I told her what I'd discovered through my online research.

Her response was defensive. I was okay with that. This time, I wasn't accepting the menopause diagnosis. We booked an office visit. Within seconds of her examining me, she agreed with my research and referred me to a specialist. Not before I broke down in tears in front of her. It served no purpose to blame anyone, but I needed to get across to her how, if my doctor had taken the time to listen to me four years earlier, they could have spared me this grief.

I will tell you what talked me off that despair ledge the night I dove down the Dr. Google rabbit hole: finding people online openly talking about their condition and what was working for them. I scoured the web for any personal reference to lichen sclerosus. My heart filled with gratitude for those with the courage to speak up. With no apparent cure (in fact, the information online loves to mention this detail, as do many members in online support groups), it seemed up to those who had LS to take up the torch. And we're doing just that. In the thousands!

By the time I saw the specialist, I'd already been using many of the tips shared online. I'd joined a vulvar lichen sclerosus Facebook group with over 5,000 members supporting each other and sharing resources. I went into this diagnosis feeling scared and alone. I came out surrounded by community. You are NOT alone in this.

In this book, I will tell you my personal story of diagnosis, treatment, and the physical, mental and spiritual practices I use to manage lichen sclerosus while continuing my research towards its origin and healing.

My journey will not be your journey. And there will be elements of LS that are not covered in this book. There is, however, a myriad of resources included here for you to continue your own investigation of LS. My intention in writing this book is to talk you off that ledge of hopelessness, anger, frustration, and despair that I not so fondly remember when I realized I had LS, and to inform and inspire you on your healing journey.

I wasn't on that ledge for long because I found support, healthcare professionals, and practices that quickly put me on the path to healing. With a 20-year background in personal training, women's wellness, nutrition, yoga, and meditation, I was well-equipped to develop a plan of treatment. It is equally frustrating, however, to feel as though you've made good choices in your life, are educated on wellness and the conditions of disease, and still end up with LS.

It's not your fault. It's lichen sclerosus and you can heal the stress of it.

ONE

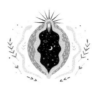

THE LOWDOWN ON LS

Whose Vulva is That?

Waiting can be the hardest part. It takes time to get in to see someone knowledgable about vulvar health, no matter where you are in the world. However, you don't have to sit idly by, feeling helpless. While I waited for my appointment with the specialist, I used what I had available: aloe vera from the plant outgrowing its pot in the corner of the tub. Fresh aloe soothed me immensely during the week I researched what else to do. I scraped fresh gel from the leaves and applied it morning and night.

Gluten was next. I'd been gluten-free during seasonal detoxes over the years, but I decided to drop the gluten for months, even a year, and see what effect that had on my body. Both of my children experienced reflux and poor sleep when they were little. After many doctor visits and sleepless nights, I pulled gluten and dairy from their diets. Their sleep improved, as did their meltdowns. Inflammation had kept them in discomfort.

My research really began at that point. After reading some posts online, I moved from using aloe vera to olive oil after each bathroom visit, since that seemed a popular solution on the web. I kept a tiny jar of oil tucked behind the plant on the tub's ledge. I applied a small amount all over each time I used the bathroom. Irritation had subsided considerably by this point and I felt as though I was moving in the right direction.

I started to think back over the years of misdiagnoses. All of the complaints that had been written off as menopause. I'd not treated anything as I never knew there was anything to treat. To compound things, I had a cervical spinal injury at age 44, just prior to menopause. I was so focused on healing the spinal injury that I paid little attention to the fact that my body needed extra support with menopause.

As I think back even further, I believe LS has always been part of my life. It just stayed at bay during my peak hormone years, popping up once in a while to puzzle doctors. Once menopause arrived, it became hard to ignore this condition.

What is Lichen Sclerosus?

From Liberty Women's Health:

Lichen sclerosus (LS) is a benign, chronic, progressive condition affecting the skin of the vulva, which is characterized by severe inflammation, changes to skin thickness (thinning or thickening) and hypo-pigmentation (loss of pigment), scarring down of the vulvar tissues such as the clitoral hood, and loss of vulvar anatomy (including partial or total resorption of the labia minora) if left untreated.[1]

From the Royal Women's Hospital, Australia:

Lichen sclerosus (said 'like-en skler-oh-sus') is a skin condition that makes patches of skin look white, thickened and crinkly. It most often affects the skin around the vulva or anus. It can be itchy, painful and cause permanent scarring.[2]

Raredisease.org has this to say:

Lichen sclerosus is a chronic inflammatory skin disorder that most commonly affects women before puberty or after menopause. Although rare, it can also be seen in men. When found in males, the disease is known as balanitis xerotica obliterans.[3]

You'll probably see references to the term *rare* a lot with LS. I don't know if I'm in agreement with this classification. Yes, I'd never heard of this condition until I went looking for my symptoms, however, a lot of people are surfacing with this diagnosis. So, I checked on the criteria for this label. Here's what genome.gov has to say:

A rare disease is generally considered to be a **disease that affects fewer than 200,000 people in the United States at any given time**. [4]

That could be true. I suspect, however, it is "rare" because it is misdiagnosed. In an online menopause group, a member complained of pain with sex and "my vagina is closing." While many members jumped in with links to vaginal atrophy and "It's normal in menopause," I was reminded of when my doctor misdiagnosed me. There's ignorance around LS because it is little-known and because it is often awkward to discuss with others, including your doctor. That's changing, thanks to all the people who are speaking up and sharing their experiences and wisdom.

According to The Royal Women's Hospital in Victoria, Australia:

Lichen sclerosus **affects around one in 80 women**. It can happen at any age, but is most common in middle-aged and elderly women.[5]

Research suggests that the most probable cause of lichen sclerosus is an autoimmune reaction in genetically predisposed individuals.[6]

Let's break it down further. Healthline says:

Lichenification is **when your skin becomes thick and leathery**. This is usually a result of constant scratching or rubbing. When you continually scratch an area of skin or it is rubbed for a prolonged period of time, your skin cells begin to grow.[7]

Sclerosus according to Miriam Webster:

I : **pathological   hardening   of   tissue especially from overgrowth of fibrous tissue or increase in interstitial tissue** also : a disease characterized by sclerosis. 2 : an inability or reluctance to adapt or compromise political sclerosis.[8]

I could have edited out the last part of that definition of sclerosus, however, I believe the mind/body connection is important in healing, and find it fascinating that the definition includes "an inability or reluctance to adapt or compromise." I know that's one of *my* psychological issues. Is the body also experiencing an inability to adapt to changes: whether through food, environment, stress, virus/bacteria or other causes?

It's important to note that not everyone experiences itching and that according to The Centers for Vulvovaginal Disorders Lichen Sclerosus Webinar[9], inflammation occurs at the basement layer of the vulvar skin. This raises the question: Is thickening due to scratching/repeated abrasion or other causes?

Root Cause and Remission

I often see the word remission in our LS groups. I'll take remission but the Scorpio in me is always seeking the deeper truth. I want a cure. Not a drug or surgery. I want to know the root cause. If we understand the root cause, we can stop the condition. Or can we?

Initially, I wondered if LS was a condition of modern times: plastics, pollution, industrial farming practices, processed foods and additives... the usual culprits of today. Or, perhaps, driven by a particular toxin (say, arriving around the time of DDT). When I pulled on that thought, it quickly unravelled. No root there.

Lichen sclerosus (LS) was described for the first time in **1887**. Since then, many synonyms have been in use, notably 'Kraurosis vulvae,' 'vulvar dystrophy,' 'white spot disease,' and 'lichen sclerosus et atrophicus' or 'guttate scleroderma.[10]

So far, the root cause is more like a root soup and each person's ingredients are unique. On the long grocery list of possible items, the LS soup appears to include any number and combination of these ingredients:

1. Hormone imbalance (low estrogen)
2. Autoimmune disorders
3. Bacterial, parasitic, fungal infection at some stage of life (reports of borrelia: Lyme disease). I had amoebic dysentery in my 20s
4. Food intolerances or allergies, leaky gut
5. Genetic predisposition
6. Issues processing oxalates or histamines
7. Physical, mental or emotional trauma (for me, this is the least understood and the factor that correlates with "inability to adapt" mentioned above)

A 2017 article in Clinical Advisor had this to say about other autoimmune issues:

The exact etiology of lichen sclerosus has not been ascertained; however, evidence points to an increased likelihood of an autoimmune and genetic component. In a study of 350 women with lichen sclerosus, researchers found that 21.5% had 1 or more autoimmune-related diseases, 21% had a family history of autoimmune disease, and 42% had autoimmune antibodies. The most common autoimmune diseases associated with lichen sclerosus are autoimmune thyroiditis, alopecia areata, vitiligo, and pernicious anemia.[11]

Just because you have LS, doesn't mean you have or will develop a second autoimmune condition. As far as I know, LS is my only one. For those of you who have already been diagnosed with an autoimmune condition, it can be comforting to know that you're not alone in this double diagnosis. I see it reported in our online support groups.

What's in a diagnosis? There is education and information, community and a common treatment protocol. But, don't be too quick to identify with your diagnosis. Continuing to tell the body it is sick, or allowing the victim to become the dominant archetype in your life has little benefit. There is an imbalance in the body/mind/spirit. **Regardless of what popular medicine names it, the goal is the same: Restore balance.**

From Mild to Severe

When my son was born, the nurses gave me 'popsicle pads' – sanitary napkins with a bit of water added to them and then put in the freezer. Let me tell you, those pads were pure heaven for relieving the pain of childbirth. I used them again after my daughter was born. That time, I added calendula water to the pads to speed healing.

Pushing a person out of your body causes substantial pain, inflammation, tearing and burning. But at least you get this adorable little human to take home with you, and once you heal, the pain does not return until you have another little human.

While comparing the discomfort of lichen sclerosus to childbirth might seem extreme, some people with LS experience excruciating pain that returns again and again. Others, myself included, are fortunate to experience mild to moderate symptoms.

What are the Signs and Symptoms of Lichen Sclerosus?

Cedars-Sinai identifies the common symptoms that may be included with LS:

- Vulvar itching (very common)
- Anal itching, bleeding, or pain
- Pain during sex
- Skin bruising and tearing
- Blisters
- Easy bleeding from minor rubbing of the skin
- Pain or bleeding when having a bowel movement
- Trouble urinating or pain with urination[12]

The challenge is that each person experiences LS differently. I suspect there can also be other issues happening alongside LS that may not be due to LS.

There was a poll posted in one of the online LS communities asking about the top symptoms experienced by its members. These were the top 10 signs and symptoms as listed by group members:

- Itch
- Burning sensation
- Redness
- White patches
- Fusing (architectural changes)
- Paper cut-like sores
- Inflammation
- Painful sex
- Shooting nerve pain
- Swelling

The list was actually 25 items long and included other items such as blood blisters, frequent urination and throbbing pain. Again, we see a soup of ingredients and not all of them may be LS related.

What are the Symptoms of Lichen Sclerosus in Children?

It saddens me to think that little ones are dealing with this condition and how challenging it must be for a parent or caregiver to figure out.

The symptom list for children varies slightly from the previous list from Cedars-Sinai. According to The Royal Children's Hospital Melbourne, these are the main signs and symptoms of LS in children:

- Itchiness
- Constipation (due to painful cracks in the skin around the anus)
- Pain when urinating
- Red and inflamed skin at the beginning, that later looks like white, shiny, wrinkled or thickened patches [13]

How do you know if it's lichen sclerosus?

There are other causes for vulvar itching. This is the complex part. Symptoms may or may not be due to LS. There may be no LS involved at all, or there may be LS alongside non LS-related issues. A specialist will diagnose lichen sclerosus from a biopsy or a visual inspection.

Since vulvas are kind of like snowflakes, no two are the same, it can be challenging for your family doctor to spot changes. It's important for you to notice changes and report them to your physician. Ask to see a specialist.

A Date with the Doctor

My GP's clinic called. "A gynaecologist has accepted the referral, but he's a male and we see here that you've requested a female. Do you want to go ahead with this appointment?"

"Shoot." I sank into my chair. *Why is this so hard?* "I'd prefer a female. I don't want to have to wait any longer though."

"I understand." The receptionist gave me the name of the specialist. "Why don't you take the day to think it over and then call us back?"

"Thank you. I appreciate that." I was already looking him up online before I'd ended the call. He delivered babies at the hospital where my kids were born. He had good reviews from patients. *Let's see what else I can find. Oh, here's his clinic.*

It turned out he is part of a dermatology clinic that specializes in vulvar disorders, specifically LS. What are the odds of that? I trusted I was in good hands. I called back and accepted the referral. You'd think the three-month wait would have been hell, but I got to work.

I did so much research on the subject that I believe my conversation with the GYN was as fascinating for him as it was for me. At least I'd like to think so. I'm pretty sure he didn't. He knew what he was looking for and immediately diagnosed me with lichen sclerosus. It was two days before my 50th birthday. Worst. Gift. Ever.

When he asked me my expectations for treatment, I told him I wanted two things:

1. To stop any further structural changes to my vulva
2. To reverse the changes if possible

I didn't know that the second thing had ever been achieved by anyone on record. I hadn't gotten that far in my research and kind of didn't want to. I preferred to at least open the door to the possibility of complete healing and reversal.

The GYN wrote me a prescription for Triamcinolone topical steroid ointment, told me to book an appointment with the clinic's pelvic floor therapist and a follow-up appointment with him in two months. I thanked him and left his clinic feeling hopeful.

Neither of the two pharmacies I tried could fill the prescription for ointment. They had only the cream. Not the preferred form, which I learned later was due to the alcohol content in the cream base which may irritate broken skin. I called the dermatology clinic and they checked with my GYN who said to go ahead with the cream. I filled the prescription.

While Triamcinolone is recognized as having a lower dose

of steroid than the typically prescribed Clobetasol propionate, I wasn't keen to use it. My daughter had experienced two years of challenging rashes that began on her hands. As the doctor attempted to treat her with various steroid creams, the rash quickly covered more of her body.

Eventually, I took my daughter to a naturopathic doctor who advised getting her off the steroids and tested her for food sensitivities. She had many. The naturopath worked with her on healing her gut and skin.

After watching her journey with steroid creams, I wanted to exhaust natural solutions before using the topical steroid on my vulva. Keep in mind, when I asked the doctor how advanced my LS was, he said on a scale of one to ten, ten being severe, I was about a two. I'm not sure if he said that to make me feel better. I experienced little irritation at this point and with the prescription filled, felt comfortable exploring alternatives. I tucked the white box into the cabinet under my bathroom sink.

Corticosteroids

This is the recommended treatment for LS. Topical corticosteroids are prescribed to reduce inflammation and itch, slow the progression of disease, stop the scarring and decrease the risk of cancer. Have the conversation with your healthcare specialist. There are varying strengths of steroid ointments/creams they can prescribe depending on the severity of your LS.

My investigation continued in online groups and I next read about ozonated olive oil in an LS thread on Reddit. My local health food store happened to carry it and that was my next step. For five weeks after my appointment, I applied ozonated olive oil each morning and before bed. I keep it in the fridge. I think it smells like high elevation hiking. My daughter says it smells like cucumbers. I used plain olive oil between applications. Any remaining itch or irritation resolved completely during this time. After being misdiagnosed years earlier and doing nothing for my vulva, giving it attention proved promising.

Controversial Borax

I found an LS group on Facebook that promoted borax soaks as a line of treatment. After another round of research, I purchased a box of 20 Mule Team Borax from my local grocery store in the laundry aisle and decided to ease into this practice. I was skeptical about this one. If it didn't resonate with me, I could always use it in my laundry.

One thing I know is that if I am fearful of a treatment, the stress alone will cause me grief. I need to feel nourished by my treatment. My qigong teacher, Master Chunyi Lin, once told us to charge our medicines with healing energy. I find this is a powerful practice if I don't feel comfortable with a particular treatment. Infuse it with love and healing intentions. Rather than feed the body fear, nourish it with blessings.

I did find interesting information about boron in the body assisting calcium and magnesium from leaching out through the urine. There is a difference, however, between boron and borax. Foods that are high in boron include avocados, prunes and prune juice, and bananas. I picked up a bottle of organic prune juice. It seemed like something to have on hand in case of constipation anyway. It's important to move the bowels regularly. More on that later. I had no interest in adding prune juice into my day on a regular basis.

While no research identifies fungal infection as the cause of LS, could fungal issues be at the root of itch and irritation for some with LS? And does that itch/scratch cycle then exacerbate LS symptoms? Why does borax give relief to some with LS? Why coconut oil? Why was aloe vera gel from the plant so effective for me in the beginning when I didn't know what else to use? All three have antifungal qualities. They are also anti-inflammatory in nature.

I mentioned LS being a soup of ingredients and while some of those ingredients are trauma, genetics, and hormones, other factors contributing to the mix (seasonings, if you will) may be more superficial like bacteria and fungus. Itch and irritation lead to scratching which, in turn, leads to broken skin, scar tissue... and on and on we go. Back to the baths.

You will see borax come up in your research. Mountain Rose Herbs has this to say about this powdery white mineral:

Borax acts as an emulsifier, natural preservative and buffering agent for moisturizers, scrubs, and bath salts. Borax is a natural mineral which is widely used in the cosmetic industry. Since it is also utilized as a detergent, many people are surprised to learn that it is also a main ingredient in their favorite bath salt.[14]

A 2018 article on Healthline states:

Borax exposure can irritate the skin or eyes and can also irritate the body if inhaled or exposed. People have reported burns from borax exposure to their skin.[15]

I will not make any recommendations for treatment. I am not a doctor nor do I play one on TV. Your protocol is between you and your healthcare team. Once again, I say this book is intended to inform you about lichen sclerosus, not diagnose or treat. The body/mind connection is powerful. It is important to feel both informed and nourished in your treatments, not fearful. You decide how to proceed with borax.

TWO

THE ROAD TO HEALING

My New Best Friend

How strange to have an informative conversation about lichen sclerosus and pelvic floor health while lying on my back, naked from the waist down, with a woman whose finger was inside my vagina.

I considered the oddness of it, then decided to relax and be grateful for her 35 years of expertise and wisdom. Honestly, I learned more from this pelvic floor therapist than the gynaecologist and felt more comfortable with her.

"Your tissues look really healthy." She stood at the foot of the treatment table. "Let's check your muscle tone. A little pressure on the left side."

I looked at the ceiling, not sure where to focus my attention. Skylights let a generous amount of natural light into the small room. "This is a really nice space." I wasn't making uncomfortable small talk. It actually was a lovely clinic. How nice to not be in a dreary clinical environment.

"Yes, we just moved into this building in March." She

shifted position. "A little pressure on the right side now. We wanted a clinic where all of us could be easily accessible to patients, rather than having to refer people here and there."

"I was shocked and grateful to discover such a clinic exists. Dermatology, pelvic floor therapy *and* gynaecology under one roof. Impressive. And needed." I noticed a footprint on one of the ceiling beams. Must have been a construction worker. It's funny where the mind wanders.

"Your right pelvic floor muscles have atrophied." She removed her finger. "It could be due to your spinal injuries. We'll follow up with that." She washed her hands and began to assemble resources for me.

She gave me samples of creams and lotions and taught me how to massage the vulvar tissues to improve elasticity. She recommended that I use CeraVe® instead of olive oil because CeraVe contains ceramides. Then she asked me about my sex life.

"I see a lot of women with this condition who have simply resolved to no longer have sex. And I ask each one the same thing." She sat on the chair across from me. "Wouldn't you at least like to have the *choice* to have sex again?"

"Of course," I responded. This conversation made me feel as though there was more than just hope for recovery; there was an actual course of treatment.

She opened her laptop and searched for resources I could explore at home. I took pictures with my phone of the websites she pulled up.

She even showed me a container of what she said is the best natural lubrication for sex: Sliquid. I bought a bottle when I paid for my appointment. I'm divorced. Still considering becoming a Buddhist nun... but you never know...

Ceramides, Lotions and Oils

What are ceramides? According to a November 2021 article in *Today*:

In short, ceramides are lipids (fatty molecules) that are found in the topmost layer of the skin to function as a barrier to protect the skin and help lock in moisture.[1]

On October 25, 2020, Healthline had this to say:

Ceramides are made up of long-chain fatty acids that link with other important molecules to promote cellular function. Ceramides **help create a barrier to prevent permeability**. This locks moisture into your skin, which helps prevent dryness and irritation.[2]

Years of working with plant oils informed me that jojoba oil would be the most natural option since it is considered the closest to skin's composition and is reported to be high in ceramides. More expensive than Cerave®, but I already had a bottle of it at home. I did appreciate the free samples and added them to my supply of salves and lotions under the bathroom sink. If nothing else worked, I'd circle back to the samples.

As an aside, sweet potatoes are considered a rich source of natural ceramides by nutritionists. I include yams and sweet potatoes regularly in my diet, especially since menopause. They are versatile and provide fibre, vitamins, and minerals (a note here to be mindful if oxalates are problematic for you).

For the next five weeks, until I saw my GYN for a follow-up, I used the jojoba oil once a day for the vulvar tissue massage and then made a concoction for bedtime. When my daughter struggled with what doctors assumed to be eczema, I'd bought every ointment, salve and balm under the sun. Needless to say, I have an expensive collection of emollients under my bathroom sink. I blended some of a pricey ointment with a comfrey salve before bed. I bought them... might as well use them.

I'd found the Facebook LS group and started taking one to two baths per week with magnesium salts, some baking soda and I even tried a little borax. What I noticed was the lines where the tissues had fused. What was once a smooth skin surface was now marked with a slight red line indicating the lost labia's edge. I got pretty excited about the prospect of unfusing, not attached to the outcome, simply hopeful.

Members in the Facebook group reported using a variety of oils, lotions and creams – from coconut oil to olive oil, commercial blends, and emu oil was a popular choice. You don't have to spend a fortune. Just find what works for you.

To me, there seems to be an order to healing:

- alleviate the itch while working to eliminate any causes of itching (bacteria, fungi, yeast, diet)
- heal the tissues (abrasions, fissures, rawness)
- strengthen the skin barrier and protect the dermis
- address inflammation in the body

According to my PF therapist, topical ointments, oils and creams need to reach the deeper layers of tissue since that's where the inflammation occurs. She instructed me to massage in any lotions for at least 90 seconds to assist the delivery to those tissues

Bowel Movements and LS

Well, this is a shitty topic. This is probably the more uncomfortable place for my LS. For nearly two decades, I thought I had hemorrhoids. I think one of my doctors mentioned it or I simply decided that was the problem. It made sense: two big babies and years of weight lifting. I had no idea LS causes scar tissue around the anal area which can create fissures when bulky stools or straining happens.

Fear of pooping is real. You push and risk a tear or you wait and the pain is slow. Too much bulk is problematic. I find a gluten-free, sugar-free, and dairy-reduced diet easier on my bowels. I keep prune juice on hand (remember, it is also a source of boron). Especially for kids with LS, finding a healthy diet that allows for comfortable bowel movements is key!

1. Ensure you eat enough fruits and vegetables that agree with your digestive system (cooked may be easier to handle than raw)
2. Decrease or eliminate processed foods
3. Drink enough water throughout the day and eat healthy fats
4. Walk or move the body daily
5. Include ground flax seeds or prune juice when needed
6. Work with a nutritionist, naturopathic doctor, or other specialists to identify any food sensitivities or gut/digestive issues
7. Mind the red meat (it may be taking up space from more fibre-rich foods)
8. Relax while on the toilet (make your bathroom a pleasant environment)

And don't forget to include the anal area in your oil massage. Just make sure you don't transfer bacteria from the anal area to the vulva. Massage the vulva tissues first and then move along to the rear.

Soaking in a warm bath can assist with keeping the area clean as well as helping the tissues to better absorb topical treatments. Soak for 20 minutes, pat dry, and apply the treatment.

You **can** repair and rejuvenate these tissues so that pain no longer plagues your pooper.

Fourchette (the 6 o'clock area)

When I originally went to my doctor in 2017, it was for this excruciating broken glass pain that accompanied penetration. This was the 6 o'clock area: the bottom of the vulva, leading to the perineum. I had no idea that my body had formed a thick band of scar tissue here.

My son was born 10 days early and weighed in at eight-and-a-half pounds. I had quite the tear and the doc stitched it up. My daughter weighed in at nine-and-a-half pounds three years later and I swear the doctor braced her foot on the end of my delivery bed to pull my baby's stuck shoulders out of the birth canal. Needless to say, the doc could've crocheted a medium-sized afghan in the time it took her to stitch me up.

My body overcompensated for that tear and I had no idea about the scar tissue. I'd just have sex, tear again, deal with it, and on and on until eventually, it was too excruciating to deal with. Penetration literally put me in fight or flight as pain coursed through my entire nervous system.

Now, my 6 o'clock area not only has a thick band of scar tissue, but there's also a scar bump right at the middle as if to seal that tissue with an extra sex-preventative button. Had I known at the time that I was dealing with LS, I would have not allowed the tearing/healing/scarring cycle to continue. Not only was it hard on my body, but also on my marriage. I was increasingly in pain. No one understood what was happening or how to support me. My body was saying "No!" but I didn't know why.

I spend extra attention now on the 6 o'clock area and massage gently while soaking. That scar bump is shrinking and the tissues are regaining elasticity.

I have no interest in online dating apps, but if I did, my profile would request a partner with a below-average-sized penis. If we can't find the humour in our situation, we've lost all hope.

The Many Faces of Trauma

According to the Cleveland Clinic:

> In some cases, lichen sclerosus develops after someone has experienced trauma, such as an injury or sexual abuse. Lichen sclerosus is not a sexually transmitted disease (STD), and it's not contagious.[3]

The Lancet weighs in with this:

> ...(lichen sclerosus occurs in skin already scarred or damaged), so trauma, injury, and sexual abuse have been suggested as possible triggers of symptoms in genetically predisposed people.[4]

A 2020 article in Obstetrics and Gynecology International continues:

A well-known manifestation of VLS is the Koebner phenomenon. It is described as the occurrence of lesions at sites of injured or traumatized skin due to scratching or sexual activity. Thus, repeated trauma and irritation to the area may act as a precipitating factor for the disease. Radiation has also been implicated as one of the causal factors.[5]

Now, I'm not a doctor or a therapist, and I don't know your particular circumstances. I *do* know that to address LS, we need to consider all the possible elements involved. A 2016 study on LS published in the National Library of Medicine says:

It is assumed that trauma plays a significant role as trigger in the development of lichen sclerosus. Such traumas include scratching, friction (e.g., caused by tight clothing), occlusion, surgical procedures or sexual abuse during childhood.[6]

I found it strange when my pelvic floor therapist asked me if I remembered ever injuring my vulva as a child, like on a bike. It was an odd question and yet immediately reminded me of when I fell vulva-first onto the frame of my bike at five years old. It was *so* painful. Clearly so, because I don't have a ton of memories from that time but I sure remembered that!

I challenge the definition of trauma to include mental and emotional aspects. Years or even decades of enduring challenging relationships, unprocessed emotions or constant negative thoughts towards your body can manifest physically.

In a 2020 interview in Human Window, Dr. Gabor Maté, author of *When the Body Says No*, describes trauma as:

> "How I think about it is that if I wounded you, if I cut your flesh, the healing would involve scar tissue forming. If the wound was great enough, you'd get a big scar, and it would be without nerve endings so you wouldn't feel, and it would be much less flexible than your normal tissue. Trauma is when there is a loss of feeling and there is a reduced flexibility in responding to the world."[7]

That scar tissue and loss of flexibility on an emotional level sounds a lot like LS on a physical level. While Dr. Maté does not speak directly to LS, he has some insight into other conditions:

> If you actually speak to these women with endometriosis or fibromyalgia, these are physiological processes, but we know from science and intuition, that the mind and body cannot be separated. These people invariably suffer from severe stress.

Dr. Maté brings it back to childhood development and feeling safe to express who you were as a child:

Those stresses have to do with suppressing the self that actually began in childhood as a coping mechanism. I've known people who have healed themselves from endometriosis or fibromyalgia and even more threatening conditions through the process of deep self work with the appropriate support.

A trauma-based therapist was briefly part of my LS journey early on after diagnosis. I was surprised to discover how my nervous system had wired itself to deal with early childhood events. My therapist helped me identify some of my core beliefs formed during childhood, and provided support and therapeutic tools.

I turned to other sources of support as well. Since LS deteriorated my relationship with my body, it was important to foster a healthy connection with my vulva, not only through soaking and massage, but also practices such as creating art and journalling. I knew from past experience with my spine that I must address trauma on all fronts.

Art and Journalling

I didn't expect to feel so disconnected from this part of my body. And I quickly realized that my growing resentment and anger could add to the burden of disease. A surprising inspiration struck one day while I was crying over the state of affairs *down there*: Draw a picture.

It seemed strange yet important for me to celebrate my vulva exactly as she is. She didn't need to be perfect or symmetrical. She just needed to be healthy, and if art was the therapy of the day, so be it.

I have a chest filled with art supplies from my days of writing and publishing children's books. I got out my favourite felt pens and some fancy paper, and spread them across the kitchen table. I knew what my vulva looked like from inspections in the mirror and I recreated her visage on the page. I added a flourish of stars and quarter moons around the paper to celebrate her. To ensure I'd taken my time with this practice, I grabbed another piece of paper and created a second image with more detail.

Surprisingly, I felt much better afterward. Creating art truly is therapy. I displayed my artwork on top of my art chest for weeks, making peace with this part of me.

Journalling came easy. As a writer, most of my books began as journal entries. I've facilitated journalling as part of wellness and writing retreats for years after reading about the health benefits of writing about pain. I recently came across a similar study where people were encouraged to write about their biggest trauma. From the 2017 BBC article, Can Writing About Pain Make You Heal Faster:

Ever since, the field psychoneuroimmunology has been exploring the link between what's now known as expressive writing, and the functioning of the immune system. The studies that followed examined the effect of expressive writing on everything from asthma and arthritis to breast cancer and migraines. In a small study conducted in Kansas, for example, it was found that women with breast cancer experienced fewer troublesome symptoms and went for fewer cancer-related appointments in the months after doing expressive writing.[8]

The article continues with some interesting insight:

Kavita Vedhara from the University of Nottingham and her team in New Zealand took 120 healthy volunteers, and made them write about either a distressing event or how they spent the previous day. They did this either before or after a punch biopsy on their upper arm. The people from the expressive writing group were six times more likely to have a wound that had healed within 10 days than the people in the control group.

I found this particularly of interest since many with LS receive punch biopsies to diagnose or follow up on their condition. Some complain of severe pain after biopsy while others have little pain at all. Expressive writing could be a useful tool to help you before your biopsy.

My journaling practice is most effective when I write exactly how I feel, where I feel it in my body, and don't censor myself. I write my fears, my hopes, my frustrations and the nature of the pain. I do this over a few days and begin to see my mood lighten quite quickly. Any time I'm plagued by difficult emotions, I take pen to paper. Then I recycle or burn the page.

This is one of the best practices I know to keep from bottling up my emotions. If you're concerned about getting stuck in the negativity, follow up your trauma with a list of all that you are grateful for. I also find that taking a walk in nature afterwards is good for the soul and for letting go. Dance, sing, shake it off and repeat as needed.

· · ·

STRESS

Sit

Tight &

Resist

Eating

Something

Sweet

As I mentioned in the section on LS causes, it's a soup of ingredients and each person's experience is unique. Within the online communities, however, there is one thing we tend to share as an LS trigger: Stress. While I enjoyed coming up with the stress-antidote acronym above, this issue goes deeper than we think.

We have an interesting relationship with stress. We throw that word around as often as we do the word *busy*. Perhaps they're related. Let's break it down.

According to the Cleveland Clinic, stress is natural:

Stress is **a normal human reaction that happens to everyone**. In fact, the human body is designed to experience stress and react to it. When you experience changes or challenges (stressors), your body produces physical and mental responses. That's stress. Stress responses help your body adjust to new situations.[9]

The stress response helps us to adapt and grow. It fosters resilience. But, what if we're stuck in a stress response?

Dr. Gabor Maté shines a light on stress and the body. From his website:

Emotional stress is a major cause of physical illness, from cancer to autoimmune conditions and many other chronic diseases. The brain and body systems that process emotions are intimately connected with the hormonal apparatus, the nervous system, and in particular the immune system. [10]

I have experienced, over my years of back pain, just how emotions can *lodge* in the body. Through writing, art, movement and even crying, ranting or chanting, these same emotions can dislodge, creating physical freedom.

There are many types of stress. We tend to think of those kind that create emotional and mental challenges: work, relationships, finances, health, etc. Then there's stress on the body. My spine reminds me every time I carry too many groceries or become overly exuberant with pilates, and it takes me longer to recover.

A deeper stress is one we cannot see: oxidative stress or OS. This stress happens at the cell level and involves our ability to deal with free radicals in the body. LS and OS are in a relationship together. And it's not going very well. According to a 2019 National Library of Medicine article:

It appears evident, as in other chronic inflammation processes, that OS plays an important role not only in the pathogenesis, but also in the development, maintenance, and progression of LS.[11]

Here's some interesting research that has me rethinking stress and LS. The article continues:

The presence of an oxidative imbalance in the diseased tissues can thus contribute to destroy the tissue of the skin and mucous membranes during LS.

Let's continue to pull on this thread...

Sander et al (2004) found that the following were present in LS lesions: products of lipid peroxidation in high concentration in the keratinocytes of the epidermal basal cell layers; oxidative DNA damage in all LS lesions; oxidative protein damage in the areas of dermal sclerosis...

What's lipid peroxidation got to do with it? I may be way out on a limb here, but it feels like this branch is connected to the lichen sclerosus tree. This next research from the National Library of Medicine (2005) is not related to LS but came up in answer to my question of how to heal/prevent lipid peroxidation (since that's what was found in LS lesions):

A combination of vitamins C and E (ascorbic acid, tocopherol) or solitary supplementation with vitamin A (retinoic acid) prevented lipid-peroxidation.[12]

Even though the focus of the research above was not LS, it appears to address a major component of the previous article on lichen sclerosus:

OS, through lipid peroxidation, is likely the most significant cause of tissue damage and consequent fibrosis, which, as the disease progresses, causes its late complications. OS is, therefore, (an) integral part of the disease and has an influence on its progression, including its possible malignant transformation.

I am sharing what I find as exciting bread crumbs (gluten-free, of course) on the path to healing LS. Including vitamins C and E or vitamin A appear to be of benefit in treating LS. According to the research included here, addressing OS is key. **I'll let the article wrap it up:**

Considering the role that OS plays in LS, therapeutic use of antioxidants, therefore, appears to be rational and possible, in association with other types of treatment. The purpose of this treatment option is not only that of reducing the damaging effects of OS on cells and tissues, but also of hindering the progression of LS and reducing the risk of malignant transformation.

It is important to work with a professional in order to get the right combination of vitamins/minerals for you, as well as dose, timing and delivery system.

It doesn't, however, mean we can't improve our consumption of foods containing these antioxidants, along with using topicals rich with them, as part of our nourishing protocols. Have the conversation with your health care practitioner.

It's interesting how, in the online groups, some people report success with eating more keto-type foods while others find relief from a lifestyle leaning towards vegetarianism. If we look at the vitamin C and E combination, we see plant-based foods such as seeds, nuts, fruits and vegetables. If we examine the keto foods, we see fatty fish, meat, eggs and dairy: all sources of retinol (vitamin A).

Perhaps it's less about the "diet" and more about the antioxidants. When we understand which nutrients we need to nourish ourselves and prevent or repair oxidative stress and lipid peroxidation, we can plan our meals accordingly. I talk more about food in the next chapter.

Of course, more research is needed.

This is only one piece of the LS puzzle, however, we need all the pieces in order to put it together. If we can't yet prevent or cure LS, perhaps we can address each of the major factors involved.

I've mentioned gut health as being another piece of this puzzle. We can also look at cellular health and address the oxidative stress in our tissues and the mental/emotional/physical stress in our lives. **It's all connected.**

I had no idea when I began writing this section on stress that I would end up talking about OS and antioxidants. And to think... I was going to tell you to breathe. Actually, I'm still going to do that but I'll make it a separate section.

So, stress really is about **S**it **T**ight & **R**esist **E**ating **S**omething **S**weet. Instead, opt for foods high in antioxidants.

Inflammation and Depression

Just when I think I can't get any more vulnerable than talking about my vulva... I will admit that depression has been an interesting invisible friend during my life. How and when it came and went often eluded me. Until my second spinal injury, six years ago, when I saw its arrival clearly, and realized an important connection. It wasn't one invisible friend who visited, it was two. Inflammation and depression often travel together. The experience had such an affect on me that I wrote about it in *Awakening on Purpose: Trusting the call:*

> It took depression less than a week to set up
>   camp. It was an odd darkness, not one that
>   came from lack of sleep or pain. It seemed a
>   foreigner who fed off the inflammation
>   ravaging my cervical spine. My world went
>   dark.
> "I've worn this outfit every day this week," I
>   said to Tanya as we sat on the park bench
>   waiting for our kids to get out of school.
>   "One thing. That's all I have the energy for.
>   One thing per day. Apparently putting these
>   clothes back on is it." I sat looking forward
>   while she sat to my right. Turning my head
>   was out of the question.

While part of our depression accompanies the diagnosis of LS, another part may be playing out without our knowledge. A 2019 article on The Role of Inflammation on Depression and Fatigue has this to say:

Depression and fatigue are conditions responsible for heavy global societal burden, especially in patients already suffering from chronic diseases. These symptoms have been identified by those affected as some of the most disabling symptoms which affect the quality of life and productivity of the individual. While many factors play a role in the development of depression and fatigue, both have been associated with increased inflammatory activation of the immune system affecting both the periphery and the central nervous system (CNS). [13]

While my cervical spinal injury was more of a one-way highway: injury causes inflammation which leads to depression and fatigue, I also wonder if that road can change directions: depression and fatigue create inflammation which leads to further injury. Addressing inflammation and all its causes, once again, appears to be a priority in management of disease, including LS.

It's not necessarily that we have a higher inflammatory load than others, but that our response is altered. It took me six years to reestablish safety in my nervous system after my cervical spinal injury. It was one of the first things I got to work on once I'd processed the diagnosis of LS.

What About Breath?

I taught meditation for years and heard many participants comment about how difficult they found it to meditate. Meditation can feel challenging, but I'll tell you what I told my clients: **The gateway to meditation is breath.**

According to the National Library of Medicine:

Diaphragmatic breathing is relaxing and therapeutic, reduces stress, and is a fundamental procedure of Pranayama Yoga, Zen, transcendental meditation and other meditation practices. Analysis of oxidative stress levels in people who meditate indicated that meditation correlates with lower oxidative stress levels, lower cortisol levels and higher melatonin levels.[14]

You caught that, right? "...meditation correlates with lower oxidative stress levels." I mentioned the role of OS with regard to LS and also the vitamins reported to help, but what about breath? What if a daily breath practice lowers your OS levels?

Breathing practice has a direct affect on the nervous system. The body is primed to balance the parasympathetic and sympathetic branches of the nervous system. Our natural circadian rhythm used to keep us on track. Today, between artificial lighting, shift-work, sleep disturbances, fast-paced and information-packed lifestyles... balance has left the building.

A 2018 article, Neuromodulation in Inflammatory Skin Disease, backs the argument for restoring balance:

Nervous system tone plays an important role in inflammatory disease, as increased autonomic imbalance has been associated with diminished response to anti-inflammatory treatment. Thus, restoration of this balance presents a potential treatment option for inflammatory disease.[15]

The article states:

The known autonomic imbalances (sympathetic > parasympathetic) seen in inflammatory disease give credence to the inflammatory reflex being an integral part of these diseases' pathogenesis...

"Sympathetic" is the branch of the nervous system responsible for fight or flight. The parasympathetic branch is responsible for our rest and digest mode. This is where relaxation and repair often happen.

Breakthroughs in the importance of parasympathetic tone in the inflammatory response have highlighted the role of the nervous system in maintaining proper immune function.

So, it would appear as though those with inflammatory disease, such as LS, spend more time in sympathetic mode (fight or flight) than parasympathetic mode (rest and digest). We can address this imbalance.

What's one method to enhance parasympathetic tone? Breath.

According to a 2018 article in CBC Life:

Breathing deeply, with a slow and steady inhalation to exhalation ratio, signals our parasympathetic nervous system to calm the body down. Long, deep breaths can also manage our stress responses to help decrease anxiety, fear, racing thoughts, a rapid heartbeat and shallow chest breathing. These responses can directly impact our physical, mental and emotional health, and longevity.[16]

Breath is powerful and available in every moment. It's also free!

Breath practice fits into *your* schedule. Choose a 20-minute practice and/or one minute of practice every hour throughout your day. I have a favourite morning and evening practice, and when my mind gets busy during the day, I take a breathing break.

One of the simplest breaths to learn is belly breathing or diaphragmatic breathing. It's also great to do with kids. According to the John Hopkins All Children's Hospital:

Diaphragmatic breathing can help in managing symptoms of chronic pain, irritable bowel syndrome, depression, anxiety and sleep disorders.

Diaphragmatic breathing assists in:
• Lowering blood pressure
• Lowering heart rate
• Decreasing levels of cortisol (stress hormone) in body
• Improving core muscle stability
• Decreasing chances of injuring muscles
• Improving ability to tolerate exercise[17]

Try belly breathing now:

1. Sitting where you are, relax your shoulders, belly and jaw
2. Put one hand on your belly
3. Inhale slowly through your nose while your belly pushes out into your hand (I tell kids it's like filling a balloon with air). Try to keep your chest still
4. Exhale slowly through the nose while you pull your belly back in (let the air out of the balloon). It might take a few breaths to get a sense of your stomach moving out towards your hand
5. Repeat for 2-5 minutes, focusing on the movement of your belly and breath together. Inhale, belly pushes out, exhale, draw belly back in

While it's good to start with a few minutes (and that's usually as long as kids can hold their attention), adults may find that working up to a longer daily practice may yield greater benefits in managing the stress of LS.

For years, I taught alternate nostril breathing. I wrote about my experience with this practice of *nadi shodhana* in my memoir, *An Accidental Awakening: It's not about yoga; It's about family*. I practiced it 11 minutes daily for a year. It had a profound effect on my mental/physical health, though it took a while for 11 minutes to not feel like an hour. I include it as a core practice in my book *Nourish: Ayurveda-inspired 21-day Detox*.

Breath continues to be one of the best things I do for my mental and physical health, including my pelvic health. I mentioned earlier the importance of adding a great pelvic floor therapist to your support team. Well, the Canadian Physio-therapy Association agrees about breath:

Breath control or pranayama (breathing methods) have long been used in yoga and can be used to downregulate the nervous system. Abdominal-Diaphragmatic breathing and Alternate Nostril breathing (Nadi Shodhana) can both be used to decrease tension in the pelvic floor.[18]

Yet another reason to commit to a breath practice to help heal the stress of LS. Honestly, between increased anxiety, worry, sleeplessness and oxidative stress with lichen sclerosus, switching into parasympathetic mode (rest and digest) through breathing practice offers a boon of benefits and a wellness practice for life.

Of course, if you create 10-30 minutes each day to allow yourself to really sink into a practice, I believe you'll find the benefits increase. Put on relaxing music, close your eyes and practice five minutes of belly breathing right now. Allow the shoulders to drop and the breath to deepen as you practice.

My guess is, you'll feel so good after that you'll create the time each day. Try belly breathing lying on your back with a pillow under your knees. Sink into your bed or the floor, wherever you practice. Inhale and your belly slowly rises. Exhale and pull your belly gently in. Soooooooo restorative.

You're welcome.

THREE

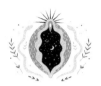

FROM FOOD TO FASTING

Food Sensitivities

I just met with my nutritionist last week for my follow-up appointment. You will hear a lot about food sensitivities and LS. You will hear about low oxalate diets, paleo, juicing... Honestly, as a former personal trainer and someone with over 20 years in the fitness/health industry, what to eat and when to eat has never been so confusing.

You'd think that with all the choices available to us, all the research and expertise, we'd have this piece figured out. But there is more stress involved in choosing and eating food than ever! What I wanted was someone to take some of the effort out of dealing with meals. I'd removed the gluten, limited dairy and dropped the sugar. Now, I needed someone to take me back to the basics and give me the building blocks to heal my gut, nourish my adrenals and thyroid and remove the guesswork and stress work out of meal planning.

I found a nutritionist who works with me on balancing blood sugar levels throughout the day, and introducing foods slowly so we can assess how my body responds. Her philosophy is not promoting a lifetime of limited foods, but healing the body so a variety of foods can be enjoyed and allowing the body to receive the majority of its nutrients from whole foods.

My philosophy is to remove the foods that give me trouble or cause inflammation in the body until I can heal my systems. Then, bring back a balanced diet. Preparation is as important as the type of food.

Soaking, roasting, grinding and other techniques are used to help with digestion and absorption of nutrients. Eating simply and seasonally is beneficial. Your attitude towards food is important. We *choose* to feel nourished. Working with a professional who has experience with autoimmune conditions can be a great addition to your health care team.

My nutritionist has me making meat stock. Not my favourite, but I live in Canada where it's cold much of the year, so meat stock feels nourishing. There is also an emphasis on healthy fats. I make simple changes and notice how I feel as I do so.

LS and Diet

If you have a history of eating disorders or find the subject of diet (by diet, I mean the foods we eat to nourish ourselves) not supportive for your journey, please skip this chapter. There are many outlets available to help you manage your LS. You do not need to contribute to your burden of stress. Work with a professional nutritionist and therapist should you wish to pursue dietary therapies for LS.

For me, landing on a nourishing diet for LS seems to involve a process of **reducing inflammation, healing the gut, eating nutrient-dense foods (including healthy fats) and balancing my blood sugar**.

In this chapter, I'll cover the foods that many with LS reduce or avoid. Paying attention to these foods in your diet and how they affect you, may help you manage your LS symptoms.

Keep in mind that one diet does not fit all. It's important to address your unique constitution, your body's needs and stressors, along with imbalances in gut health. Sometimes, people discover they have sensitivities to certain foods, and once eliminated, LS symptoms abate. Work with your doctor, naturopath or nutritionist to help identify any allergies/sensitivities and improve your gut health.

It's all connected. Your body is this beautiful orchestra. The organs are the instruments and sometimes they get out of harmony. With some care and attention, we can guide them back towards balance.

It's not about making food your enemy. It's about finding what nourishes you. Make one change at a time and keep a journal to record any differences you notice. What happens when you eliminate sugar or gluten? How do you feel when you gradually reduce high-oxalate foods like spinach or high-histamine items like alcohol?

Intermittent Fasting

According to Johns Hopkins Medicine:

Intermittent fasting is an eating plan that switches between fasting and eating on a regular schedule. Research shows that intermittent fasting is a way to manage your weight and prevent — or even reverse — some forms of disease. But how do you do it? And is it safe?[1]

The article goes on to say:

There are several different ways to do intermittent fasting, but they are all based on choosing regular time periods to eat and fast. For instance, you might try eating only during an eight-hour period each day and fast for the remainder. Or you might choose to eat only one meal a day two days a week. There are many different intermittent fasting schedules.

I find that it's less about following a program and more about discovering your ideal eating routine. I use intermittent fasting as a way to balance my blood sugar levels throughout the day. Some people choose to eat two large meals a day. That doesn't work for me. Eating too many calories in one sitting creates stress on my system.

I've noticed that I do well eating about every 3-4 hours during my window. So, that's what I do. Please note, there are currently no studies on lichen sclerosus and IF specifically. Nourishment is a personal journey.

In my book *Nourish: Ayurveda-inspired 21-day Detox*, one of the practices I suggest is to not snack after dinner. My clients reported benefits like better sleep, weight loss (if indicated), improved digestion and mood (once you get past the evening munchies addiction). This is a practice that has also worked for me.

I slide my dinner time a bit later, finishing by 7:00pm, so I'm not hungry by bedtime (10:30 - 11:00pm). And I like to eat breakfast between 9:30 and 10am. That gives me a fasting window of 14-15 hours and an eating window of 9-10 hours. This works for me. Find what works for *you*.

Can intermittent fasting heal the gut?

The next sections on sugar, gluten and dairy focus not only on the foods themselves, but on healing the gut. This is an issue that comes up again and again with autoimmune disorders. This is what the Cedars-Sinai blog has to say:

We've done studies looking at the effects of doing a single fast by looking at changes in the gut microbiome (the collection of microscopic organisms—including bacteria, fungi and viruses—that lives in our bodies) and markers of inflammation in the gut in mice. We also studied healthy humans to look at the gut microbiome to see how it changes with 2 fasts per week. At the 12-16 hour mark, we saw a dramatic shift in the gut microbiome population after fasting for that period. Certain bacteria are super responsive to fasting, and those tend to be beneficial bacteria. The concept is that with intermittent fasting, you could permanently grow those bacteria and experience the associated benefits.[2]

That's fascinating. A change in how and when we eat can potentially improve our good bacteria and our overall gut health.

How long before I know if intermittent fasting works for me?

The Johns Hopkins Medicine article answers this question:

Mattson's research shows that it can take two to four weeks before the body becomes accustomed to intermittent fasting. You might feel hungry or cranky while you're getting used to the new routine. But, he observes, research subjects who make it through the adjustment period tend to stick with the plan, because they notice they feel better.

That's the biggie. "They notice they feel better." This is what I read in the LS online communities for those who have tried IF. When you start to feel better, you want to continue feeling better, so you are motivated to continue with your nourishing IF ritual.

Who shouldn't try intermittent fasting?

The Johns Hopkins article advises:

Williams stresses that before you try intermittent fasting (or any diet), you should check in with your primary care practitioner first. Some people should steer clear of trying intermittent fasting:
- Children and teens under age 18.
- Women who are pregnant or breastfeeding.
- People with diabetes or blood sugar problems.
- Those with a history of eating disorders.

Talk with your health care practitioner to see if IF is a good fit for you. If you're not sure where to start, often eliminating your evening snacking is enough to feel better in your body. Ensure you eat enough nutrient-dense foods in your day.

Sugar-free

When I was little, every Easter I'd get one of those giant chocolate bunnies. Well, giant is relative, I was little. I would break off its ears in delicious anticipation, take one bite and then promptly stuff the disfigured bunny back into the box and under my bed. Eventually, Mom would get mad because it would attract bugs. We lived on a farm.

I make no apologies for stuffing that waxy, sugary, tasteless chocolate under my bed. I am a chocoholic and have been for most of my life. However, for me, chocolate, good chocolate, is like herbal tea: high vibrational, nutrient-dense medicine from Mother Earth (it is, however, also high in oxalates).

Sugar is not my issue. I don't like hard candies. I don't drink pop. It's not that I never have sugar but I certainly notice when I do. In fact, managing my blood sugar levels is one of the best things I do for both menopause and LS.

So, what's sugar got to do with lichen sclerosus?

I believe that gut health is the key to good health. And sugar plays a big part in this mystery. According to Dr. Suhirdan, Gastroenterologist and Hepatologist:

Too much sugar can reduce beneficial bacteria, leading to a leaky gut syndrome. An increase of pathogenic bacteria, which is the species of microorganisms that cause diseases, can lead to a condition known as dysbiosis. An increase of this type of bacteria causes changes to the internal mucosal barrier of the intestine.[3]

The Sydney Gastroenterologist goes on to say:

There are up to 1000 species of bacteria in an individual's gut microbiome. Bacterial cells in the body outnumber human cells by around 10 trillion. While most species are beneficial to our health, certain species are the cause of diseases.

If there is a possibility that bacterial, parasitic or fungal infection play a part in aggravating LS, it would seem important that we do our best to ensure not only a healthy gut lining but also a happy gut microbiome.

How do we do this? Rather than pumping probiotics on top of the bacterial gut party, we first need to remove the fuel for the bacteria we don't want. Reduce the sugar and those unwanted partiers will move along. (Okay they'll die off, but that sounds like a tragic way for a party to end).

Gut health and children with lichen sclerosus.

A pilot study published in the National Library of Medicine in 2021 looked at LS in kids as it relates to the skin and gut microbiota. The study had this to say about the results:

In the gut samples, girls with LS had a significantly higher relative abundance of Dialister spp., Clostridiales spp., Paraprevotella spp., Escherichia coli, Bifidobacterium adolescentis, and Akkermansia muciniphila, and a lower relative abundance of Roseburia faecis and Ruminococcus bromii compared to controls. These results suggest a potential association between cutaneous and gut dysbiosis and pediatric vulvar LS.[4]

That's a pretty big deal. We know that our gut health and our immune system are connected. I believe we can begin to address autoimmune conditions, including LS, by paying attention to our gut health.

One more note from the Sydney gastroenterologist on how long it takes to improve the gut biome:

Depending on how extensive the effect of sugar on gut bacteria was, the gut microbiome could take some time to improve. That being said, the average time it takes to build up a healthy gut microbiome is about 6 months.

There is no quick fix when it comes to regaining your health. It is, however, a journey worth taking. Reducing sugar is another promising step along your LS road to health. Again, it's not about labelling a food good or bad; it's about figuring out what's nourishing for you at this time.

And it's not your fault. It's not as simple as what you've eaten in the past. There's nutrition, inherited biome, overprescribed antibiotics, farming practices, soil depletion and food production on a global scale... it's a whole ball of wax (and you know how much I dislike eating wax). I can't change the whole system right now. What I *can* do is make simple nourishing choices each day.

Keep packaged products at bay. Eat a whole foods diet. Enlist the support of a nutritionist or discover nourishing sugar-free recipes online.

If you need to wean yourself (or your kids) off sugar, opt for honey, pure maple syrup or fruit. Though I do still buy chocolate, I've been making my own for over a decade. That way, I choose the ingredients: no wax, no refined sugar. And it never ends up under my bed.

Gluten-free

According to the Gluten Free Society:

There are a number of triggers for autoimmunity... a simple overview of these triggers:
- •Foods (gluten, dairy, processed sugar are common)
- •Chemicals (pesticides, heavy metals, plastics, etc)
- •Nutritional Deficiencies (vitamin and mineral inadequacy)
- •Microbes (viral, bacterial, fungal, parasitic)
- •Intense prolonged stress
- •Genetic predisposition[5]

The list above sounds familiar: many of the same causes I listed for LS. I'm not going to get into the gluten debate. It makes no sense to make something our enemy. The goal is to remove any foods that may be adding to your burden of inflammation, then heal your body with nourishing additions. **It's not about focusing on what you can't have, it's about adding more nutrient-dense foods that nourish your unique needs.**

Before my diagnosis of LS, my spidey senses told me to eliminate gluten, not just for 30 days, but for six months to a year and see what happens. After the first three months, I could hardly believe how flat my belly felt. No bloating or sluggishness. Constipation was rare. Oh, and I stopped snoring, which had become a thing during menopause. As hormones decline, inflammation can increase.

Note: Don't rely on packaged gluten-free products. Replace gluten with whole foods: vegetables, fruits, meats and healthy fats.

Dairy-free

I used to think yogurt gave me yeast infections. It was supposed to be the other way around: yogurt was meant to be good for getting rid of yeast infections. I love yogurt. But if I have it for more than two or three days, itchy irritation sets in.

Once diagnosed with LS, I realized it wasn't a yeast infection that yogurt triggered, it was LS. Either dairy didn't work for me, the probiotics in it weren't the right ones, or the higher histamine levels in yogurt were at play. We'll talk histamines in the next section.

I'd stopped drinking milk years ago when my kids were little and dairy triggered digestive issues, plugged ears and snoring for them. And then I just got used to a milk-free diet. I found butter agrees with me, so I keep it on hand for its nutritive and delicious properties. I also enjoy the occasional soft cheese.

Dairy is also a piece of my menopause snoring puzzle. Like the Bermuda Triangle of foods, gluten, dairy and sugar are a mysterious force and where I find my snoring at its worst. When I reduce/eliminate those ingredients, snoring goes away.

I'm not telling you that dairy is at the root of your LS, I'm encouraging you to get into a conversation with your body. Get curious about what you eat and why. Notice what nourishes you and what may no longer be nourishing you at this time.

Work with a nutritionist or do some personal investigating. **Keep a journal**. It's easy to forget from day to day how we feel. Note the date, what you ate, when and where (were you at the kitchen table listening to Mozart or wolfing down lunch in your car?). Then, note anything of interest: sleep, bathroom habits, physical and emotional changes. No more snoring?

Don't get caught up in micromanaging your diet. Take a relaxed, investigative approach with your food. If you choose to eliminate dairy for a couple weeks or more, bring it back in slowly. Notice any changes.

Remember, there's no need to label a food good or bad. Don't blame the food. It could be that dairy isn't great for you during the cold winter months but agrees with you in the summer. It could be that other things are creating a burden of inflammation in your body and dairy is tipping you over the edge. It could be the histamines at play rather than the yogurt.

Oxalates

One of my favourite foods as a kid on the farm was rhubarb. Strawberry/rhubarb pie, rhubarb jam... put rhubarb in it and I'm here for it. One of the first things we learned as kids on the farm was not to eat rhubarb leaves. No one explained the chemistry. We didn't care to know. Just that the leaves are toxic. Nuff said. Go play in the stinging nettles behind the barn.

What makes rhubarb leaves toxic? A high concentration of oxalic acid. Great insect deterrent. Not great for people.

I've covered gluten, sugar and dairy in the previous sections. Now, let's look at another common complaint I see with LS and food.

What are oxalates? According to a Urology of Virginia article:

Oxalic acid or oxalates are very tiny molecules that bind minerals like calcium and form crystals. It is found in a variety of seeds, nuts and many vegetables. 6

So, what's the issue with oxalates? The article continues:

Oxalates not only can cause kidney stones (calcium oxalate kidney stones) but also may be responsible for a wide variety of other health problems related to inflammation, auto-immunity, mitochondrial dysfunction, mineral balance, connective tissue integrity, urinary tract issues and poor gut function.

There are reports of those with LS finding relief by following a low oxalate diet. My focus is to figure out why certain foods don't agree with my body and address any underlying issues so that I can enjoy a variety of good foods.

Before we go blaming foods high in oxalates for our troubles, let's read on to discover a familiar key mentioned in the sugar-free chapter. I won't pretend to understand the complexity of oxalates and the body.

Having a damaged gut lining will increase your absorption of oxalates. An inflamed or damaged gut lining is a very common problem, thanks to frequent antibiotic use and the presence of a number of chemicals in our food supply, including glyphosate. Other plant compounds such as phytates and lectins (such as gluten) can worsen gut health and exacerbate the impact of oxalates.

It's not so simple, is it? We return to gut health and the gut lining. It's not about getting rid of oxalates. It's finding out why some bodies can't deal with them. According to the Restoration Healthcare website:

Oxalates aren't necessarily a cause for alarm. You may be able to eat foods high in oxalates without experiencing any health issues, while someone else — because of how their body processes oxalates — needs to be careful about what they eat. Because of our bio-individuality, our systems handle micronutrients and anti-nutrients differently.[7]

This rabbit hole led me to Sally K. Norton, who has an impressive list of credentials and experience with oxalates. She has more to add to the oxalate debate. She tells us that along with getting oxalates through our foods, our bodies make it and:

Some fungi make it, possibly for mineral management, especially in soil

1. Can be made by Aspergillus fungi living in the body.[8]

Along with gut health, one of the other issues I come across with LS is mineral imbalance. Two peas in an autoimmune pod, I suspect.

According to my nutritionist, removing oxalates from your diet in one fell swoop can cause what's known as *oxalate dumping* and a temporary worsening of symptoms. So, work with a professional or take your time in reducing these foods.

I've tried dropping chocolate cold turkey and let me tell you, there's a lot of pain involved. Ninety per cent of it is emotional.

Oxalates and vulvar pain.

According to the Vulval Pain Society:

Dietary oxalate consumption does not appear to be associated with an elevated risk of vulvodynia.[9]

The Hoffman Centre for Integrative and Functional Medicine, however, says oxalates can irritate the vulva:

Vulvodynia/interstitial cystitis and benign prostatic hypertrophy (BPH). Both these conditions cause chronic pain in the vulva, which can be unbearable for female patients that are afflicted. Vulvodynia is a misunderstood disease, which was linked to oxalate by the late Dr. Clive C. Solomons. He identified that high levels of oxalate can irritate the epithelium of the vulva and cause pain if there was prior trauma in the area. Oxalate aggravates a pre-existing condition, but also irritates the glycosaminoglycan layer in the bladder.[10]

You see... quite the rabbit hole. Before you identify oxalates as your issue, remember to not blame food. There's a lot more involved than ingredients.

It's not just about what we eat, but how we prepare our food. Soaking and then rinsing nuts and seeds can decrease the total oxalate content. So can boiling and, to a lesser extent, steaming our food. Rather than expect our digestive system to work for us regardless of what we pump into it, we need to prepare food that assists our system in nourishing us. Let's help our guts out.

Histamines

We want to pick out one thing and say, "That. That is the cause of my LS." And by removing that cause, we heal. It doesn't appear to work that way. Everything is connected. There is an entire system involved.

When I began to manage my blood sugar levels, I noticed a reduction in hot flushing and fatigue. I balance my blood sugar not only through food but also by not over exercising, stressing or overthinking (yes, that's a thing for me. My busy brain burns a lot of fuel).

According to Dr. Becky Campbell:

It's often overlooked yet there is a strong connection between histamine and your blood sugar. Research has shown that blood sugar imbalances can increase your histamine levels. Stabilizing your blood sugar is an absolutely critical aspect of improving histamine intolerance and MCAS symptoms. [11]

s is actually what triggered me into diving deeper into ﹍ ﹍﹍ histamines. I came across a study that suggested there were mast cell granules in lichen sclerosus biopsy samples.[12] What were the mast cells trying to accomplish?

Mast cells and histamines.

From the Healing Histamine blog:

Mast cells, and the histamine they release, are first responders in times of infection. It's believed that mast cells recruit neutrophils and other immune cells, and take them to places where autoimmunity is causing destruction. This activity results in an intensification of localised inflammatory response, causing and sustaining tissue damage.[13]

Keep in mind that some of this comes back to gut health. The gut usually keeps oxalates and histamines in check. If you choose to experiment with a low oxalate/low histamine diet, remember, the end game is a healthy gut.

According to Dr. Ruscio's 2020 article entitled *Everything You Need to Know About Histamine Intolerance*:

One study suggested that inflammation and intestinal permeability (leaky gut) caused by bacterial imbalance were likely involved in histamine intolerance. Another study showed that 30%-55% of people with digestive symptoms also have histamine intolerance. Bacteria produce histamine, so an overgrowth of bacteria contributes to histamine load.[14]

As I mentioned in the section on oxalates, how we prepare our food has a lot to do with how we digest it. This holds true for histamine in the diet. The National Library of Medicine has good info on this:

Grilled seafood had higher histamine levels than raw or boiled seafood. For meat, grilling increased the histamine level, whereas boiling decreased it. For eggs, there was not much difference in histamine level according to cooking method. Fried vegetables had higher histamine levels than raw vegetables. And fermented foods didn't show much difference in histamine level after being boiled. [15]

One of the well-known symptoms of histamines is itching. Many other symptoms accompany histamine intolerance, but that's one symptom that LS sufferers deal with a lot. Seek a nutritionist or professional to assist you, or keep a food diary and notice if histamines play a part in your LS.

In feeling empowered to manage our own symptoms of LS, how and what we eat helps put management into our own hands. Exploring our connection to food is a worthwhile endeavour. For our individual health and the health of the planet.

Taking the Sting out of LS

I dug around my pantry looking for the bag of nettles I'd bought months earlier. Sometimes, a plant just speaks to you and you pick it up, not even knowing what it's for. I found the bag and made a strong cup of tea.

During my journey, I decided to raise awareness for LS by blogging about one component of this condition each day for a month. I had no idea how much more I would learn about LS during my month of writing. You know the expression *All roads lead to Rome?* Well, I discovered along the way that all of my LS research was leading to nettles. Perhaps those roads have ditches lined with these wondrous plants often considered weeds.

You see, as soon as I realized that nettles are antihistamines, I added the tea back into my day, hoping to drive down inflammation in my body. And then I found the research on oxidative stress and the vitamins involved in prevention/remediation: A, C, E. Guess what nettles have?

And then there's the oxalates issue. One of the recommendations for dealing with oxalates is to increase calcium intake. Dr. Lani Simpson, Certified Densitometrist and Bone Health Expert says:

If prepared correctly, nettle tea is high enough in calcium to be considered an aid in bone-building. Some of the other conditions it may help include insomnia, osteoporosis, arthritis, adrenal depletion, skin conditions, indigestion, low iron and even headaches.[16]

And nettles are low in oxalates. It's the perfect plant, provided it's the right medicine for *you*. Remember that LS is a journey unique to each of us. Some people report nettle allergies.

And boron? Shut the front door. In a 2018 National Library of Medicine research article, *Urtica* spp.: Ordinary Plants With Extraordinary Properties:

Urtica (nettle) leaves in addition contain **boron**, sodium, iodine, chromium, copper and sulfur [17]

Are nettles too good to be true? As with any herb, It's important to work with a professional.

A 2018 Healthline article, 6 Evidence-based Benefits of Stinging Nettle, advises:

Pregnant women should avoid consuming stinging nettle because it may trigger uterine contractions, which can raise the risk of a miscarriage. Speak to your doctor before consuming stinging nettle if you're taking one of the following:
- Blood thinners
- Blood pressure medication
- Diuretics (water pills)
- Diabetes medication
- Lithium [18]

Know how to best consume them. Stinging nettles have prickly barbs that you want to avoid. Trust me. As kids, we often encountered them while playing behind the barn. Fresh nettles can cause irritation. **Don't consume the fresh plant.**

It is best dried, cooked or purchased from your local health food store. You can buy it as a tea, tincture, capsules and even a cream/topical. Or grow your own. Nettle soup, anyone?

FOUR

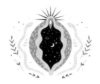

SUPPORTING THE VULVA

The Hormone Conundrum

The follow-up appointment with my GYN arrived. I expected another physical examination. This time, I was met by the head resident from the hospital my GYN works at. She was there to discuss hormone replacement therapy with me since I'd mentioned it at my first appointment. That was to be our next step.

After a long conversation with her about types of HRT and finding the best one for me, she left the room to ask the GYN a question for which she didn't have the answer. My GYN returned with her and answered my question about HRT; more importantly, he answered my question about whether or not it would help with the LS. He said no. Basically, it was just for my hot flashes and sleep issues. So, is LS an estrogen-deficient disease or not? Research suggests there could be an implication, though the consensus is that HRT does not improve LS.

I mentioned that I had yet to use the steroid cream he'd prescribed. While I know steroids are the recommended treatment, I wanted to experiment first with some of the things I'd discovered in my research. He did admit that other than steroid creams, he really had nothing more for me. It was now between me and my pelvic floor therapist.

It's challenging enough to deal with LS as an adult, I can't imagine our children dealing with it. The GYN asked if I have a daughter, and told me this is a conversation I'll have to have with her. While I don't believe she has any vulvar LS active symptoms, skin rashes have bothered her for years. Once her diet and gut clear up, her skin issues also tend to clear, though not always.

I would never advise you to not use what your doctor prescribes. I will say that the majority of my healing over the years has come from "alternative" sources. For me, they're not alternative, they're natural. I'm grateful for modern medicine and our access to it. I do believe that taking a holistic approach offers the best outcome for healing. And how great it is to have freedom of choice.

The bottom line for me is, as always, trying to find the root of this condition and a nourishing way to manage it long term (if not heal it completely). Community and conversation are key, a sense of humour is a must and some thick skin (pun intended) is helpful. If nothing else, we shall attract much-needed attention to vulvovaginal health.

HRT

I filled my prescriptions for HRT after my GYN follow-up and headed home. I was excited and nervous about starting hormone replacement therapy. A month ago, I was hopeful it was the answer to my sleep issues, my hot flashes and my LS.

I read the enclosed pamphlets for the prescriptions and became scared, frustrated and confused. My mom is on HRT with no side effects. I know many are, but I can't get my head around it. I just don't want to take estrogen and progesterone every day. I know, I know, don't read the comments online. But I did. I can't unread them. So many complaints of headaches, nausea, bloating, bleeding and mood swings.

Yes, I crave deeper sleep and a healthier vag, but I don't currently have any of those other symptoms and if taking HRT gives me them, I don't want it.

Sometimes I feel as though I need to stop trying for perfect health and simply agree to be happy with where I am. Stop pointing a magnifying glass at what's wrong and celebrate what's right. Honestly, that's what my heart keeps telling me. Find a nourishing routine. I'm good enough. Done.

But what if the HRT allows me to sleep like a baby? What if the side effects are non-existent because it's the right medicine for me at this time? What if it stops the LS? Research shows this not to be the case and my GYN agrees, but every person is different.

A March, 2022 article in the National Library of Medicine reported a study on LS using topical progesterone cream vs Clobetasol for 12 weeks in premenopausal women. At first glance, Clob is the victor. Good news for Clob.

What's interesting is this statement:

"LS was in complete remission in 6 out of 10 patients (60%) with available biopsy in the progesterone arm, and in 13 out of 16 patients (81.3%) in the clobetasol propionate arm". [1]

That's a high remission rate... for Clob *and* for progesterone cream.

Great news on the LS treatment front. If I had it my way... that study would have been on Clob vs. Triamcinolone vs. progesterone cream vs. estriol cream vs. estradiol cream and including pre and post menopausal populations. Then I feel like we'd covered most of our bases.

My LS symptoms have been few lately. Some kind of moisturizer (I've used many) is key, along with the salt baths and I have no complaints. Other than the fusing. I have hopes to reverse some of that. So, do I really need HRT for menopausal symptoms? I can talk myself in and out of it depending on the day. It's a personal choice. And thank the goddess for the choice. It's one more element (and conversation to have with your doctor) along this LS/menopause journey.

What Triggers a Flare?

I hadn't even thought of this term until I joined the Facebook group. Members use it often. I haven't experienced flares in the way others talk about them: sudden increase in pain, cuts, tearing, unbearable itching, boils... though that could have been happening during my years of misdiagnosis. My experience is more: Whose vulva is this? Treatment. Daily maintenance. Stop stressing over it. Focus on my healing practices. Managing well.

What I *have* noticed over the years, keep in mind I've dealt with spinal injuries and pain off and on for almost two decades, was that after a period of stress, I'd crash. When I moved houses last year, I pushed through the packing and cleaning out the old house while prepping the new one. Once I'd moved into the new house, I could barely move my body. No particular areas of pain or discomfort, just complete fatigue and fog. The autoimmune component made sense once I realized this. Or, it could have been rampant inflammation.

So, what triggers a flare?

This is for LS to know and you to find out. Everybody is different. I know you want to discover your triggers so that you can manage this condition yourself. Here are some common causes and questions to ask of your health care team:

1. Food sensitivities, oxalate dumping
2. Contact allergies (underwear, detergent, soap, even toilet paper)
3. Stress
4. Gut health
5. Lack of sleep
6. Reaction to the medication
7. Vitamin/mineral deficiencies
8. Hormone fluctuations

Illness can also trigger a flare, though I tend to find the opposite is true for me. When I get sick, other pains in my body disappear. It's as if the immune system (and also my mind) actually have something to work on so they stop focusing on my spine and vulva!

Pelvic Floor Therapy Follow-up

I had a follow-up appointment today with my pelvic floor therapist. I love her. She says my tissues look amazing and that my pelvic floor muscles have improved and she wondered why my GYN doesn't have me on a topical estrogen cream to soften the scar tissues and plump. So... get this... she texted him during our appointment to recommend a cream for me. She felt a topical estrogen cream for the vulva/vagina would be of greater benefit than full HRT. She said that since the vulva tissues look healthy, we're moving on to stretching the tissues at the entry of the vagina.

Here's the interesting part. She explained how the tissues need to move in different directions (like they do with sex) and that with LS and the scarring, they no longer do. Because of this, regular dilators are not the best tool to begin with. She got out a massage wand and said that the tissues at the entrance of the vagina need to be massaged and stretched dynamically.

It's definitely worth including a PF specialist on your care team. Mine told me that the patient she saw before me had come for her follow-up and was finally able to insert a tampon for the first time in her life! If we want to empower ourselves to improve the effects of our LS and vaginal atrophy, pelvic floor therapists have a wealth of knowledge and techniques to share with us.

She said to use a tiny amount of the steroid cream just on the scar patches a couple times a week and also use the topical estrogen cream once I get it. The PF therapist did say that topical estrogen creams can mask the LS symptoms.

In Search of the Lost Labia ... A Vulva Adventure

It was not easy to sort through all the research on estrogen creams. I wanted to know more about topical estrogen before choosing this route of care. I also wanted to know what to do about fusing and loss of architecture. Could I recover more of my lost labia?

This is a complex issue and a conversation to have with your GYN, dermatologist or functional medicine provider.

Labial adhesions: topical estriol cream. This particular study involves *children* with labial adhesion (different from LS and menopausal atrophy; however, it seemed to apply similar treatment protocols).

Many physicians offer young girls estrogen cream to be applied on the labia for several weeks to treat labial adhesion. While no randomized controlled trial data are available, the success rate of such creams is reported in the literature to be close to 90%. Side effects of estrogen cream are mild and transient. Although the ideal frequency and length of treatment with estrogen cream have yet to be determined, most treatment recommendations suggest an application of the cream 1 to 2 times a day; treatment should be applied for a few weeks before considering surgical alternatives.[2]

Menopause alone can bring structural changes to the vulva. Topical estrogen creams are used to assist in slowing or even reversing these changes. From Harvard Health Publishing:

Estrogen cream and other vaginal estrogens are very effective treatments for atrophic vaginitis, a condition that's common in postmenopausal women and results from a drop in estrogen levels. Estrogen loss can lead to thinning (atrophy) of the cells lining the vagina and urethra. As a result, women may develop vaginal dryness, itching, and pain with intercourse, as well as a high risk of urinary and vaginal infections.[3]

Again, it's worth a conversation with your doctor as to whether this is a good choice for you. Estrogen therapy is not recommended for everyone. When I returned to see my GYN, he agreed with my pelvic floor therapist that topical estrogen cream would be of benefit to me.

What About Cancer?

I know it's easy to say don't worry. It's harder to do. Worry has never solved anything. I don't brush off the increased cancer risk, however, I certainly don't make it my focus. This is between you and your doctor to stay on top of. It is also one of the reasons to find and develop a spiritual/wellness practice. More on that to follow.

If you've read my other books, *An Accidental Awakening: It's not about yoga; It's about family*, or *Awakening on Purpose: Trusting the call*, you'll know that I've spent the past 20 years managing spinal issues. Just when I think I've healed everything, I come back to realize that healing can be a life-long process and that the body guides us to create a nourishing environment for ourselves.

There was a point in my life where there was no doubt in my mind that I would heal completely. There have also been many times that I'm grateful I can walk with friends, play *Just Dance* with my daughter and get out of bed in the morning. Because in the back of my mind, in criss-cross applesauce, sits the possibility that one day all that could change. My spine could fuse, nerves could continue to compress and loss of motion could set in. But not today. Today, I meditate, listen to Jack Johnson's uplifting music, make nutritious meals, write, enjoy a walk with a good friend and hold the intention for continued healing.

Anything can happen. We cannot worry about *anything*. We can, however, continue to create nourishing rituals and routines, practice healing and happiness, and participate in the conversation around LS.

I now do visual checks weekly on my vulva (mainly because I got really excited about the unfusing and want to continue to cheer it on). Plus, my response when I first saw it months ago in its unrecognizable state was severe. Now, it looks so good that I enjoy continuing to improve my relationship and response to this part of the body that receives little attention until something goes wrong.

Monthly checks are probably fine. I don't stress about every little bump. I make mental notes of any changes and know that I can discuss them with my specialist when necessary. The great thing about the pelvic floor therapist is that I see her monthly for a while, so I feel like I have someone to discuss changes with, especially early on in this diagnosis. The GYN will see me annually for checkups, however, I've got my PF therapist to have these conversations with in the meantime.

Still, cancer repeatedly comes up in conversation in the online LS groups. Of course, we'd love some piece of research to tell us it won't happen to us, but no one can say what life will bring. We can listen to the experts, perform regular self-exams along with visits to the doctor, fine-tune our intuition and do our best to care for ourselves and those around us.

The increased risk of cancer among those with LS is reported by various sites to be between 3-6%. So, let's first put that in perspective. I would hazard a guess that chronic worrying is more harmful to our health than a 3-6% increased risk of vulvar cancer. That said, it is not my intention to disregard it. It's one more reason to take better care of ourselves.

Early research did not support long-term steroids as a cancer preventative. According to an article on Cancer Therapy Advisor:

While topical steroid therapy is clearly beneficial in terms of symptom control, there is little evidence that its long-term use or optimal control of symptoms reduces the risk of malignancy. Because lichen sclerosus confers an increased risk of vulvar malignancy, long-term follow-up is required. Persistent or suspicious lesions (e.g., ulcerations, masses) should be biopsied in order to exclude intraepithelial neoplasia or invasive squamous cell cancer.[4]

A 2004 study posted on JAMA Dermatology had this to add:

Although a protective effect from malignant evolution is suggested (carcinoma developed only in nontreated or irregularly treated VLS lesions), the number of seemingly protected patients was too small to be statistically significant.[5]

As much as I wanted to find a study that proved steroid treatment wasn't needed to prevent the possibility of cancer, when I posted the above in an LS online community, the group administrator provided me with the following updated study:

A study of 507 women, of which 357 adhered to treatment with topical corticosteroids (compliant) and 150 did not carry out the advised treatment (partially compliant).

> There was a significant difference in symptom
> control, scarring, and occurrence of vulvar carcinoma
> between compliant and partially compliant patients. [6]

The above study showed that 4.7% of those who didn't use topical corticosteroids as prescribed or used them irregularly, developed precancerous cells or carcinoma. We understand that using no treatment increases the risk, however, how about those using acupuncture/TCM, naturopathic remedies, PRP injections, herbs or other treatment protocols? The 4.7% is in line with the 3-6% increase reported by various sources.

The good news is... according to the study above, treatment appears to be effective. It just doesn't agree with every person. An article on Cureus has this to say:

> The side effects of TCS include irritation, burning,
> dryness, hypopigmentation, and dermal atrophy. The
> adverse effects of stinging, burning, and dryness are
> most commonly due to the base of the topical steroid
> rather than the steroid itself; hypopigmentation and
> dermal atrophy may occur with topical steroid use,
> particularly to keratinized skin, but these side effects
> are specifically noted to rarely occur in most long-term
> studies of topical steroids for treatment of VLS.[7]

What has fuelled my investigation of LS, beyond this mysterious condition itself, is my desire for an effective treatment that doesn't involve a lifetime of steroid use. While I'm grateful for access to modern medicine, I'm curious about other treatment approaches.

Let's add one more stat to the conversation. According to the American Cancer Society, the five-year survival rate for vulvar cancer (all stages combined) is 71%.

Women now being diagnosed with vulvar cancer may have a better outlook than these numbers show. Treatments improve over time, and these numbers are based on people who were diagnosed and treated at least five years earlier.[8]

When we take all of this into account, yes, LS is reported to increase your chance of vulvar cancer by around 3-6%. That's already low. On top of that, those who *do* develop vulvar cancer have at least (improving with time) a 71% five-year survival rate. The research showed 86% for localized cancer.

There are members in the online communities who have had surgery or minor procedures to remove cancerous areas. And they report doing well. There are far more who are cancer-free. And, according to the study mentioned above, conventional treatment appears to be successful in eliminating cancer risk from LS.

I can't tell you what to do. This is why LS (really, most health issues) is such a personal condition. Have the conversations you need to have with your health care team and make the choices that are best for you.

What we know is that regular check-ups are needed, self-exams keep you alert to any changes, and a holistic healing lifestyle (addressing all the parts of you and LS) helps ease your mind and support your body.

Fusing

One night, I noticed irritation. It worried me. I checked my vulva in the mirror the following morning and I saw the source of the irritation: my tissues looked swollen, especially on the right side where I felt raw. The labia had partially unfused. I had hoped for a reversal of structural changes, and had also let that go so as not to cling to any potentially frustrating outcome.

It's been four months of focused attention on vulvar care. I've been gluten, dairy and refined-sugar-free. I've had salt baths about twice a week for three months. I am not linking causation here, I'd rather ask questions.

1. Is the unfusing partly due to my mineral baths? If so, does this indicate fungal involvement in the condition or anti-inflammatory nature of mineral baths? Is it a mineral deficiency? Acidity/alkaline environment?

2. Are all the strategies (gluten-free, dairy-free, sugar-free, balancing blood sugar levels with what I eat and when, daily probiotic) reducing inflammation and sources that lead to autoimmune response?

3. How much of these changes are due to vulva massage of the tissues, both in the bath and after using oils and techniques from my pelvic floor therapist?

And the big question for me (though less of a question in my mind): how much of this is from my spiritual practice and the work I've done with healing any trauma around my sexuality, past partners, feelings about my sexual health, childbirth trauma, removing energy blocks and cultivating love for my body and self?

The 7-day Blessing at the start of the year was a powerful week of qigong practice for me. And my almost-daily (I do my best) happiness meditation continues to inform my cells and connect my body.

On day seven of the 7-day Blessing, Master Lin focused on clearing all karmic blocks to health, relationships and abundance. He mentioned that sometimes we seem to get so close to healing but it never quite happens or something sets us back, and that can be due to karma that we are unaware of. I believe this. I have believed in karma and unseen causes for some time now. It's how I live my life so it's not a stretch for me to dig into these practices.

If it's a stretch for you, I encourage you to find some form of practice that brings you joy. Maybe it's not qigong or chanting. Maybe it's gardening or your animals. While qigong and meditation are powerful, so are you. And your ability to sit with your painful emotions and have compassion for them and yourself, then choose to feel happiness and gratitude every day, will go a long way towards your healing. I believe this to be true.

Your Relationship and Sex

I know of people who have divorced because of LS and those who have enjoyed support from their partners. I know of some who simply decided sex wasn't worth the discomfort and of those who did their therapy exercises and managed to restore their vulvar health and sex life. As my pelvic floor therapist said, "Wouldn't you like to have the choice?"

My husband and I chose to divorce. We made a decision to work towards a healthy outcome for ourselves and our children. I can't blame LS. I didn't know I had it at the time of our decision, however, I'd be lying if I said it wasn't a factor. Being misdiagnosed for years probably made things more difficult.

The doctors kept calling it menopause, but since I was only in my forties, that felt like a hopeless sentence.

If we'd caught the LS earlier, perhaps emollients, massage and vaginal dilators could have slowed the progress and improved our sex life. But there's no point in pining over the past. These options are available to me now.

If you plan to use a dilator, take time to restore the skin first. Get the tissues in good condition before using dilators. Do your soaks and massage and use your ceramide oils/creams to improve the skin's elasticity. While I use a cervical wand to improve vaginal canal shortening due to menopause, I've had improvements in vulvar tissue elasticity from massage alone. Give your skin its best chance at pliability by improving the tissues first.

I entertained the idea of a monastic life and letting sex fall right off the table. But I'm not ready for that. I agree with my pelvic floor therapist. I'd like the choice. While there is so much more to life than sex, my vulva still needs healing and, honestly, great sex would also be nice. Those living with LS have many options for continuing to enjoy intimacy and arousal (with their partner or on their own). If this is an area of stress for you, consider seeking support from a pelvic floor or sex therapist.

LS or Atrophy?

Menopause at 44 seemed harsh to me. Didn't *they* say women hit their sexual prime at 42? Thanks for the generous window of pleasure. Followed by the cliff of post-menopause.

It occurred to me that LS is not to blame for everything happening with my vulva and vagina. I'm five years post-menopausal and I know my estradiol is very low (I had it measured). Some form of hormone therapy probably would've been quite restorative years ago (and even today).

I'm certain some of my changes would have happened even if I didn't have LS. What I find the most helpful, rather than blaming LS and complaining about "this terrible disease" (which I read often in the online groups), is addressing the issues. It doesn't matter if the painful sex is LS or atrophy, my course of treatment is directed at restoring my sexual health.

According to the Mayo Clinic:

Vaginal atrophy (atrophic vaginitis) is thinning, drying and inflammation of the vaginal walls that may occur when your body has less estrogen. Vaginal atrophy occurs most often after menopause. For many women, vaginal atrophy not only makes intercourse painful but also leads to distressing urinary symptoms.[9]

Burning, dryness, itching, UTIs, shortening and tightening of the vaginal canal, and painful intercourse are all cited as symptoms of menopause. What I *haven't* come across in the literature on menopause are the white patches, thickened skin, scarring, ulcers and sores on the vulva that many with LS experience. These seem to be more LS-related than menopause-related.

When I reached menopause (I wasn't aiming for it, trust me), I didn't realize just how extensive the physiological (never mind emotional/mental) changes could be. The Australian Family Physician identifies these changes due to menopause, what they term the genitourinary syndrome of menopause (GSM), and what used to be termed vulvovaginal atrophy:

> The loss of oestrogen causes anatomical and functional changes, leading to physical symptoms in all of the genitourinary tissues. The tissues lose collagen and elastin; have altered smooth muscle cell function; have a reduction in the number of blood vessels and increased connective tissue, leading to thinning of the epithelium; diminished blood flow; and reduced elasticity. Thinning is also related to the change in the vaginal epithelial cells.[10]

There's a rather big hot spot in the LS community around the word "thinning". We see it used on most sites referring to LS symptoms. We know that lichenification is thickening and that tissues become thickened with LS. There is also reference to LS appearing like cigarette paper: shiny, thin and smooth. This is my experience. So, while LS may be a condition of thickening, the appearance of my vulvar tissues is one of thinning. And, as we can see from the above information on GSM, thinning tissues can be an issue of menopause. While the medical community continues to learn more about LS and figure out this dynamic of thinning/thickening, I am focused on treating all symptoms as they arise and working towards potential root causes.

Which symptoms are from menopause and which are due to LS? Rather than get caught up in naming and blaming (do it once then move along), address the issues at hand and include the therapies that help you get where you need to go. Tightening of the vaginal canal may be best addressed by a good pelvic floor therapist. Your GYN, dermatologist or specialist will help you with changes to your vulvar/vaginal tissues and any issues with going to the bathroom or UTIs.

I believe that half of my symptoms are due to vulvovaginal atrophy or GSM, therefore menopause and low estrogen-related. Working on my adrenals, liver and gut health, along with relaxation practices, are my focus at this point. Knowing that estrogen masks the symptoms of LS (why we often don't know we have it until menopause), it is important to address underlying inflammation, gut health and stress, but if you're post-menopausal, don't be too quick to blame all of your issues on LS. Find a pelvic floor therapist or other specialist versed in menopause relief to support you.

FIVE

AN ALTERNATIVE APPROACH

Acceptance

It's funny, but I have learned deep acceptance through my divorce. I open more each day to let my ex-husband (it still feels weird to call him that; let's go with the father of my children) live how he lives during his time with the kids. I still interfere now and then around matters of their diet and health, but I've had to (no, I choose to) practice letting go and learning to accept. How wonderful it is that my children have an amazing relationship with their dad. That was my intention from the beginning of our separation: healthy relationships between us all.

And I practice acceptance around my children. They are teenagers with choices of their own and lives to live. I don't need to solve all their problems or fix the stars and planets in the sky so that their paths are always protected... as much as I'd like to. The universe loves them as much as I do.

Neither can I heal my own childhood through projection onto my children. In an attempt to ensure my wounding did not become their wounding, perhaps I held too tight or worried too much. I will never apologize for loving too much, but I will turn my attention to the one who needs the healing right now. Me. What I learn through my journey with LS, I can pass along to my daughter (and son) should they need it.

Adrenals

Winter of 2019, I pedalled as fast as I could to keep pace with the Saturday morning spin class. I'd convinced my husband at the time to join the class and said I would come along for support. Heart disease ran long and deep on the paternal side of his family: most men having their first heart attack in their 40s. Regular exercise was a key for his health, mood and winter weight gain. It was, however, the last thing I needed. I closed my eyes and dove into my inner world to conjure energy and open my channels, often visualizing ancestors or ancient ones celebrating with me in the class.

My naturopath was treating me for adrenal fatigue at the time. We'd done a hormone workup called the DUTCH test, and most everything came back low, very low. Estradiol was negligible and cortisol was nearly non-existent. Most of my hormones came back in the low range, even for post menopause.

Forward to 2022. I drove my kids' dad to the hospital. He had two stents put in. He went from having reasonable cholesterol levels in 2019 to chest pain every morning and two 70% blockages in one artery. The procedure went well, and he is back to golfing and will soon return to cycling. A part of me felt bad for not being there these past couple of years to continue supporting him in managing his health. A bigger part, however, realized that I cannot manage everyone else's health. Especially at a cost to my own.

So, what do the adrenals have to do with LS?

I've mentioned hormone imbalance as a possible cause of LS. In menopause, the adrenals become responsible for hormones. Tyson's Gynecology (The Menopause Centre) has this to say:

Additionally, the adrenal glands are able to produce **sex hormones** when their levels decline during perimenopause. However, current or built up stress can deplete the adrenal glands and inhibit their ability to boost sex hormones. As a result, adrenal fatigue can worsen a woman's menopause symptoms.[1]

When I think of the adrenals, I think of the phrase, *not enough*. Our feelings of not-enoughness cause us to push harder than we need, take on more responsibility, and run on stress. In our 20s and even 30s, our hormones happily help us recover. In our 40s and 50s however, as sex hormones decline, this stress response catches up with us and the adrenals strain under the burden. It has taken me some time to support my adrenals. Some of the things that had to go were:

1. People-pleasing
2. Trying to control or micromanage everything
3. Chasing the next thing (it might be the answer, the cure, the miracle)
4. Worrying (this is a work in progress)
5. Trying to accomplish everything
6. Prioritizing everyone else
7. Social media time (too much comparison energy and wasted time)

And more of this:

1. Accept everyone and everything as they are
2. Accept that I am enough in every moment, have always been enough
3. Let myself acknowledge that things are better than my mind likes to conjure
4. If all I get to today is making nourishing meals and spending time with my kids, that's a great day
5. Dare to be happy. Exactly as I am. Exactly as the world around me is
6. Accept that the entire universe loves me as I am
7. Put myself in high-vibe environments (nature, friends, laughter, music, movement, meditation)

The adrenals need extra nourishment in midlife. We are often managing homes, work, children, parental care and our own health. The adrenals are "on call" a lot. This is a time to heal the past, recover the present and open a door to a more healthful future. We accept all the pieces of us and where we are at this point in life. No regrets, blame or shame. Happy adrenals. Smiling adrenals. You are enough.

Manage your Energy, not your Time

I came across this phrase years ago and thought I'd adopted it. Over this past year, however, I saw how many times I pushed past hunger because I wanted to write one more paragraph or answer one more social media comment. In fact, I'm in the middle of trying to ditch social media. It's a work in progress. What does that tell us? An addiction? Yes. But why? While I enjoy the community, truth be told, I envy those who live their lives offline.

I have recently married the "Manage your energy" saying with an old Zen Buddhist saying: "Eat when you're hungry, sleep when you're tired."

I'm listening to my body and its energy needs. I'm recalibrating my rhythms (more likely they're recalibrating me), and I'm noticing when I choose to ignore these signs and excavate the reason beneath my avoidance. As much as my mind (or often our culture) wants me to live full speed ahead, my body says no. Not now. Perhaps not ever again.

I had an argument with my daughter this morning. Within an hour of our argument, I noticed a sensation along the right side of my vulva. It was as if the stress went directly to that area. I've spent the better part of this past year calming my nervous system. Implementing daily practice is key for me: qigong, meditation, nature, music... something that soothes the nerves, mind and spirit.

As I witnessed my body's response to the argument, I realized it's even more important that I manage my energy. Disagreements will happen, though I can choose to engage or not. A daily recovery plan is required. A nourishing practice of some sort restores balance. Belly breathing is often enough to decompress.

The Other G-spot: Gratitude

Nineteen years ago, I was bedridden due to a lumbar spinal injury. I had a full-time career as a personal trainer at the time. I eventually got back on my feet, married and had two awesome kids. I thought I could just go back to living my life, playing all the sports and doing all the activities I wanted. My spine had other plans. Some days, I couldn't lift my daughter from her crib. I spent years in yoga and, through complementary alternative therapies, managed to heal my back.

A second injury occurred six years ago, this time in my cervical spine, and I returned to working on healing my back. When the LS diagnosis came last year, it was another blow. "Come on, Universe! Isn't one health issue enough?!"

It took me a hot second to get my head around it, however, here's the gift of my spinal injuries:

- I am grateful every day that my body supports me
- Dancing in my living room is pure joy
- Walking with a good friend is something I will never take for granted

My injury moved me from personal training to writing books, and I've loved every minute (okay, most minutes).

LS certainly threw me back, but the gifts of the previous injury caught me and reminded me how I live slower, speak more kindly to myself and hold space for all of my emotions. I no longer pine for the past me. And I'm grateful each day. Just imagine: in our next life, we'll talk about walking around the house without any pants on and we'll laugh and laugh...

Gratitude Benefits

Mental health is as important as physical health. Often, in online communities, I read members' posts of depression over this diagnosis, anxiety over checking on the condition every day (Is it worse? Is it better?) and chronic worry over the possibility of structural changes to the vulva and the increased risk of cancer.

It is crucial to our health that we find and devote time to practices that improve our mental wellbeing and empower us to participate in our healing every day. Gratitude is one such practice. The research is in.

In a 2021 Harvard Health article entitled Giving Thanks Can Make You Happier:

...Dr. Martin E. P. Seligman, a psychologist at the University of Pennsylvania, tested the impact of various positive psychology interventions on 411 people... When their week's assignment was to write and personally deliver a letter of gratitude to someone who had never been properly thanked for his or her kindness, participants immediately exhibited a huge increase in happiness scores. This impact was greater than that from any other intervention, with benefits lasting for a month. Of course, studies such as this one cannot prove cause and effect. But most of the studies published on this topic support an association between gratitude and an individual's well-being.[2]

A 2017 article from the Greater Good Magazine states:

It's important to note that the mental health benefits of gratitude writing in our study did not emerge immediately, but gradually accrued over time. Although the different groups in our study did not differ in mental health levels one week after the end of the writing activities, individuals in the gratitude group reported better mental health than the others four weeks after the writing activities, and this difference in mental health became even larger 12 weeks after the writing activities.[3]

From the Global Autoimmune Institute:

Research has shown that gratitude can decrease stress hormones like cortisol and produce a "shift in autonomic balance toward increased parasympathetic activity," otherwise known as the "rest and digest" state. For individuals experiencing anxiety, sensitivities, and other health issues who may be operating in a chronic "fight or flight" mode, sending the body into a relaxed state can positively impact health and aid in the healing process.[4]

The practice of gratitude, along with creating art, journalling, dancing, singing... helps to shift us from a state of helplessness to a state of empowerment. There is something you can do to manage your health. Many things! You are not helpless. There's hope. In fact, there's more than just hope, there's help.

Gratitude Journalling/practice

There are many ways to include gratitude in your daily life. You can create a morning and evening practice of writing down five things you are grateful for. Be specific. Do this practice every day for a month and notice how you feel.

There's more to gratitude practice than journalling. When I wake up, I practice *feeling* gratitude before I even get out of bed. I feel grateful (yes, sometimes you have to conjure this feeling) for my bed, my pillow, the sun shining or the furnace that brings heat in a cold Canadian winter. I feel grateful for my home and my day ahead filled with choices and freedoms and possibilities.

You can FEEL grateful throughout your day, in random moments:

- While washing your hands, feel grateful for clean water
- While eating, feel grateful for your food
- When talking to friends or family, feel grateful to have these people in your life
- When looking out the window or walking outside, feel grateful to know nature, birdsong, blue sky, air, earth under your feet

Take a moment to conjure gratitude. Remember something that draws the feeling naturally to you. Then make it your practice to do so again and again. One day, you will feel it for no reason. It will become second nature to you. Life shifts when we live from this place of gratitude.

If you struggle to feel grateful, then simply invite it into your life. Pretend, imagine, be available for it. It will come. That's why we call it practice. Commit to it every day and see what unfolds for you.

This is a powerful practice to share with your children. Right before bed, take turns with each of you finding three to five things you feel grateful for that day. It's a way to discover what's happening in your kids' days and teach them to cultivate gratitude as well. Sleep comes easier to a grateful heart.

Mixed Messages

My pelvic floor therapist had commented that my right pelvic floor muscles were weak and that it could be due to nerve issues. I have a history of lumbar/sacroiliac joint issues. There may be a problem with innervation to those right pelvic floor muscles due to nerve compression or issues with the low back. While the therapist recommended an appointment with a neurologist, my doctor decided to refer me to a physiatrist: a doctor who specializes in movement, particularly after spinal injury.

Because my GYN said he sees LS occasionally accompanied by ankylosing spondylitis, I included it in my research expedition (I did eventually see a rheumatologist who believes AS is not at play for me and that my spinal issues are predominantly biomechanical, most likely resulting from my scoliosis).

One of the things I discovered in my research, however, is particularly interesting. Epstein Barr virus can be implicated in AS and other autoimmune conditions. EB was said to reprogram the B-cells of the immune system (I'd not heard that before). This makes sense from an autoimmune standpoint.

The EBV invades the B cells themselves, re-programs them, and takes over control of their functions. The Cincinnati Children's research team has discovered a new clue about how the virus does this, a process that involves tiny proteins called transcription factors.[5]

What's fascinating to me is that during the qigong 7-day Blessing, Master Lin spoke about wrong messages in the body. That the cells simply have wrong information and that during our practice, we see these wrong messages leaving the body as extra energy.

Could this wrong messaging in the body be from a variety of sources? Sources that can be measured/identified and sources that are less recognized such as:

1. Virus/fungi/bacteria
2. Ongoing trauma
3. Our internal dialogue/thoughts
4. The comments and interactions with family/friends/community (the news?)
5. Childhood and ancestral trauma/beliefs/genes
6. Past karma
7. Food/environmental toxins

Can we simply change the messaging? Louise Hay spent her life's work on that very thing. Likewise, Dr. Joe Dispenza has taken up that work. In fact, many pursue this line of thinking.

I would go so far as to say that chanting mantras throughout the day is an effective way to reprogram your cells. Feeling happiness and conjuring joy every day is a way to change the messaging in your body. Sitting in nature and listening to birdsong is a way to change the messaging in the body. Eating a diverse variety of healthy foods and herbs is a way to change the messaging in the body.

Mind your Thoughts and your Words

Last year, I experienced a subluxated shoulder. After trying to remedy it myself through gentle stretching and strengthening, I finally saw my chiropractor. While adjusting the arm, he asked me to repeat after him: "I know who I am." I repeated his words. "I know where I fit in." Again, I complied. "I know my purpose." I completed the set.

"What if I don't believe it?" I mumbled into the face cradle of the treatment table.

"Doesn't matter." He continued to work on my shoulder. "Your body just needs to hear it."

That conversation reminded me that my cells are listening. It's not about feeding my body bullshit. It won't stand for that either. It is, however, about being mindful of the messages you plant in your tissues every day.

Often I see people commenting online on this "horrible disease" or responding to someone who is now symptom-free that there's "no cure" and they're *only* in remission.

There was a time when many well-educated folks believed Earth to be flat. Be careful what you think you know and even more careful about stepping on others during their healing journey.

What's that old saying? ***The person who thinks it cannot be done should not interrupt the person doing it.***

We're not burying our heads in the sand about LS. We're doing all we can to heal it: body, mind and spirit. The gift of LS is that as you work towards a compassionate cure for yourself, you heal other aspects of your body and life along the way. And who's to say what might come from a commitment to heal? Perhaps we each hold a piece of that puzzle.

What's the Message?

Though my LS journey has felt swift since proper diagnosis, my journey through injury has been long. It has taken me some time to get to where I am. After writing *An Accidental Awakening*, I thought I'd healed my spine. Then the cervical spinal injury threw me for a loop, and I was angry.

What helped me was the realization that anger was both the root of my dis-ease and the route to my healing. I needed to deal with it. And it's taken years to walk this road. So many gifts along the way. I know people say this... but I wouldn't change it. It got me here, and here feels good.

You are living your life complete with all its messy bits. No one promised us perfect health, and I don't believe it's a marker of a life well-lived. During the worst of my back pain, I discovered a new perspective:

When pain was a daily companion, I took the words of beloved Buddhist teacher Thich Nhat Hanh, "*I have noticed that people are dealing too much with the negative, with what is wrong. ... Why not try the other way, to look into the patient and see positive things, to just touch those things and make them bloom?*" and I applied them to my physical pain.

I sat on my front step and scanned my body. It's easy, when you are in pain, to focus on the pain. This is like putting a spotlight on it. Instead, I searched my body for a place that didn't hurt — where I had no sensation. Some days that took a while. Nope, that hurts. No, that too. But eventually I'd find a spot, even if I worked all the way down to my left baby toe.

Then I would keep my full attention on that toe. Before long, I noticed my pain subsided in other areas. I found the positive and rested with it, allowing it to bloom.

Find the positive in your body or day and breathe with it. Allow it to bloom. Even if it is your left baby toe.

HOUSEHOLDER YOGINI: PRACTICES & JOURNALING EXERCISES FOR WOMEN WHO LIVE AT THE INTERSECTION OF SPIRITUALITY & FAMILY

The Science of Energy

During my spinal injuries, when doctors had nothing more to offer me for back pain other than steroid injections, I turned to complementary alternative medicine. If we open our minds to a holistic healing model, we may advance healing. In addition, we free up doctors and specialists to do the great work they do while we participate in our own healing.

We can widen our lens to include new possibilities in health. Also, the ancient yogis had little in the way of scientific instrumentation, and they had a profound understanding of the body and its systems, along with healing practices.

What *does* the science say? According to the Mayo Clinic:

While a growing body of scientific research supports the health benefits of meditation, some researchers believe it's not yet possible to draw conclusions about the possible benefits of meditation.

With that in mind, some research suggests that meditation may help people manage symptoms of conditions such as:
- Anxiety
- Asthma
- Cancer
- Chronic pain
- Depression
- Heart disease
- High blood pressure
- Irritable bowel syndrome
- Sleep problems
- Tension headaches[6]

A 2017 article in New Scientist on inflammation looks at a study by Ivana Buric, a psychologist at the Coventry University's Brain, Belief and Behaviour lab:

> The team analysed 18 trials including 846 participants, ranging from a 2005 study of Qigong to a 2014 trial that tested whether tai chi influenced gene activity in people with insomnia. Although the quality of studies was mixed and the results were complex, Buric says an overall pattern emerged. Genes related to inflammation became less active in people practicing mind-body interventions.[7]

That's a pretty big deal when we consider the role inflammation plays in autoimmune disorders. We talked about oxidative stress in the section on LS and stress. We also talked about breath and its role in reducing OS and inflammation. Tai chi and qigong are yet more tools to add to your LS holistic healing toolbox.

What does TCM have to Say About LS?

According to The Acupuncture Clinic in Hastings, New Zealand:

> **What can cause lichen sclerosus according to traditional Chinese medicine (TCM)?**
> There are a number of causes or patterns of disharmony involving a number of organs. Probably the most common pattern is known as damp heat in the

lower burner. The damp heat condition also can correlate to yeast infection and thrush and the treatment principle is to use herbs that clear heat and resolve damp.

Another common cause is due to the liver. The Liver meridian transverses through the genitals and excess heat can get trapped in the meridian and accumulate in the genitals. A weakness or deficiency in the body can also lead to the vulvar not being nourished by energy and blood and hence leading to a disposition to be invaded by pathogens according to traditional theory.[8]

That last comment is interesting. I've found great success from the pelvic floor therapy exercises I've been given. It seems as though the exercises are helping to nourish the vulvar and pelvic area tissues.

I've endured tingling down my legs and into my feet for years (and often a numb vulva from sitting or cycling too long). Since I've been doing my pelvic floor exercises and increasing the number of times I preform my qigong cupping practice on my sacrum and tailbone area each day, I've not had any tingling or buzzing/numbness. I've never been so focused on nourishing my vulva!

More Energy

Having written a book on chakras, I'd be remiss if I didn't address the energy elephant in the room: the energy centres involved in LS. From my book *Householder Yogini*:

Chakra, *Sanskrit* for wheel.

When we speak of the chakra system, we most often refer to the seven main energy centres in the body, starting from the base of the spine and ending at the crown of the head. These spinning wheels are responsible for the flow of *prana*, life force energy, through a system of *nadis* or channels in the body.

Known for thousands of years, the chakra system is most often associated with the spiritual practices of yoga or the healing practice of reiki. When the channels become blocked, dis-ease of the mind and body can follow. When the channels are clear and open, energy flows freely, leading to increased health and higher states of awareness.

The ancient practices of yoga have married with the western practices of psychology as many practitioners make connections between the physical, emotional and spiritual bodies of the individual.

As I contemplated the areas of my body affected by LS, I considered the chakras involved. The first is the root chakra (energy centre at the base of the torso: vulva and anus). More from *Householder Yogini*:

Root chakra emotional issues, like fear or feeling unsupported, can be carried through from childhood, a less than ideal relationship or a poor work environment (to name a few). These conditions chip away at our foundation over time. They shape our perspective and form our belief patterns.

After years of using myriad techniques to manage pain from a series of spinal injuries, my fear response was on high alert. I often needed to console my mind and fear response. When panic arose over pain or conditions that may increase pain, I often reassured myself, "You are okay. You are safe. It's all good. Relax." This dialogue assisted me in befriending my response and patterning rather than creating increased struggle and resistance in my body and mind.

If the body is trapped in a fear or pain response, we need to investigate the emotions that may be repressed, redirected and mistakenly expressed through the physical body. If pain or conditions of the legs, feet, knees and bottom of the torso (hemorrhoids, constipation) exist, ask yourself what emotions you are feeling.

Am I afraid of something? Is there a lack of support (material, emotional or otherwise) in my life? What are my needs that aren't being met?

Root chakra is responsible for a strong foundation, safety, security and support. Its element is earth. This is where we feel grounded. Or not. Personally, I noticed fear from my childhood trapped in my nervous system's response to life. I needed to both address that fear hypersensitivity while also using it to create a kinder, gentler environment for myself. I use myriad techniques:

1. Meditation/qigong
2. Time in nature, whether a walk with a friend or sitting in the forest
3. Uplifting/relaxing music

4. Movement such as cycling or pilates
5. Laughter, gratitude and happiness as a daily practice (and some days that practice is challenging!)
6. Letting go of what isn't important or worth struggling over
7. Herbs such as passionflower or supplements such as L-Theanine

When I find my nervous system overwhelmed, I simplify my environment. One thing at a time.

The other energy centre that comes to mind when I consider LS is second chakra.

Second chakra sits nestled in the pelvis. This energy centre is responsible for creativity, sensuality and sexuality, relationships, abundance and playfulness. It is also the seat of emotions. Its element is water.

Guilt, blame and shame reside in sacral chakra. This energy centre governs our reproductive organs. It makes sense that this centre is involved in LS.

Once we address the root chakra issues of fear, safety and feeling supported, we investigate our feelings of blame, shame and guilt related to our childhood, sexuality and relationships. This is when I turn to journalling, art and other forms of expression to help the energy here flow.

Of course, therapy can be beneficial while you speak with a professional about the traumas in your life. Even if your life has been relatively trauma-free up until now, it can be helpful to speak to someone about your feelings around LS. Receiving this diagnosis can add to your overall burden of stress. Seeking support from a professional such as a psychologist, or even a sex therapist, may reduce this burden and support your healing.

For second chakra healing, I try to incorporate the following:

1. Dance
2. Music
3. Play (with a family member, a pet, a friend)
4. Create (something, anything... gardening, pottery, snowman, poetry, knitting, good food, vulva art)
5. Deepening my friendships and choosing wisely who I spend time with
6. Oil massage for my vulva
7. Meditative soaks in the tub (often with a few rose petals or drops of essential oils)

When it comes to second chakra, it's about letting go of guilt, blame and shame, and daring to be happy– where you are, as you are.

Support Groups

The more time I spend in the LS support groups, the more I feel myself obsessing (and stressing) about LS. The same energy happens ... we get in this loop of something's wrong with us, then we continue to seek out ways to reinforce this message. It's time to change the messaging.

My morning qigong happiness meditation is a healing ritual that seems to seep through barriers and re-inform my cells that I'm not in a state of crisis. That I'm in a state of wellness. This is the mindset I practice.

One of my favourite movies is *Love Actually*. I watch it every year around Christmas. In one of the movie's storylines, the best man is secretly in love with the bride. He keeps it to himself but obsesses over her. One day, he arrives at her door with a series of cardboard signs. He flips from one to the next while she reads his confession of love, and then he agrees to let it go. As he walks away, she runs out after him and gives him a kiss then runs back inside. He continues on his way, saying to himself, "Enough now. Enough."

It's time to stop obsessing over LS. To let my body feel well again. *Enough.*

Years ago, while reading about healing, something caught my attention. I can't recall the source. You know how you come across something and it feels like a deep truth? This was one of those for me.

The author wrote about deep psychological connections to disease. That when someone starts a new therapy, they have a positive initial healing response, only to be back suffering weeks or months later. A new therapy begins with similar results and 'round and 'round it goes. This could point to the power of placebo/nocebo, however, the deeper truth that the author stated was that there was a psychological block to healing (possibly in the form of unresolved trauma).

I'm not saying LS is in your head. Never. I have it. It's definitely not in my head. Quite the opposite direction to my head. I do believe, however, that my mind has a lot to do with it. I also believe it goes further than the unresolved trauma of the individual. It could be rooted as deep as family trauma/imbalances, ancestral trauma, collective trauma or even karma.

Especially when children are involved, I question dietary, environmental, birth conditions, genetic predisposition, bacteria (the usual culprits), and I also wonder about the birthing parent's immune system/biome passed along to the child, the family trauma, birth and ancestral conditions.

Energy is information. There is information involved in disease. Oftentimes, it's misinformation– wrong messaging in the body.

With kids, meditation and healing practices may not be a therapy route of choice for them to do themselves; however, you can practice for them. Every day, I call my family and friends (and you, dear reader) into my meditation practice. I see their smiling faces behind my closed eyes and I send them all the love and healing that I practice for myself. We can do this for one another. We are all connected. Perhaps we can change the messaging together.

Qigong, meditation and self-compassion have all helped with re-patterning my nervous system. It's a daily practice. I believe disease points us in the direction of health. Some journeys are longer than others. All are worth taking. I constantly walk this line between using my illness/injuries as teachers pointing me in the direction of greater healing and helping me let go of this conditioning of "there's something wrong that needs to be fixed."

In the beginning, support groups are a God-send. You no longer feel alone. You learn a ton about which remedies people are using and which professionals to see. But, there comes a point when you go into the group and suddenly it feels heavier than before. You are outgrowing the group.

Yes, in the beginning of diagnosis with LS, it can feel anguishing and too much to bear. Sharing those emotions is helpful. Remaining in that state for too long will not improve the situation. You will move through the stages of healing. Know when *your* time in support groups is enough.

Self-compassion

Compassion is key for me. Making peace is progress for me— in more ways than simply healing from LS. LS becomes the teacher that helps me learn deeper compassion and shows me where unprocessed trauma continues to reside in my body. LS points me in the direction of deeper practice: qigong and meditation, aligning my body with mind and spirit.

Eventually, though, all roads lead to compassion. I know I still have anger to process. But I feel like I can reach compassion quicker than I used to. Rather than ask, "Why did this happen to me?" I can ask, "Why did this happen *for* me?" I've received many gifts from illness. All of them in some form of a simpler, slower, softer, lighter and happier life.

It's strange, but it's almost as if LS and I are walking alongside each other. I begin to look at it like a friend. I feel warmth towards my condition. For my spine. Even as I type this with a headache that I'm pretty sure is coming from my neck, and my son is in the basement recovering from Covid, I still feel warmth towards all of these conditions of my life. A warm blanket of peace. I think to feel otherwise would bring more mental and physical suffering.

That's not to say I don't lose my shit from time to time. F-bombs drop regularly around here. But it's reassuring to know that, more and more, I can feel at peace with life. My body and I are learning to get along again. It reveals what needs to be healed, and I turn to nature, my teachers and my practices to digest what hasn't been. Then I let go, again and again.

SIX

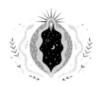

A NOURISHING RITUAL

Skipping School for Self-care

I was supposed to be on a Zoom call for a course. But, it was Sunday and I wanted to prioritize some serious self-care, LS-style. My son had homework and my daughter slept in. I emailed my absence to the group. Here's how my day began:

- Drinking warm water with lemon
- Outdoor meditation, including belly breathing
- Gluten-free, sugar-free, dairy-free breakfast
- Steeping nettle tea while I ran the tub
- Mineral salt bath with vulva massage to work towards releasing areas of fusing or scarring
- Post-bath application of topical estriol cream to assist with plumping the tissues
- Natural topical blend of oils to keep the tissues healthy
- Vulva/pelvic massage/release techniques as taught to me by my pelvic floor therapist

I took my time and enjoyed a slow morning of nourishing practices. In all honesty, it took me about 90 minutes. My daughter still wasn't up by the time I'd finished.

Some with LS have a full daily-care routine. I have a more minimal daily routine and include a longer session (like the one above) once or twice a week. You'll find or create one that works for *you*. My LS ritual keeps me comfortable and has improved the quality of my vulvar tissues.

I mentioned before that, to me, there seems to be an order to healing:

- Alleviate any itching from bacteria, fungi, yeast
- Heal the tissues (abrasions, fissures, rawness)
- Strengthen the skin barrier and protect the dermis
- All while addressing inflammation in the body

Let's talk topicals.

It's important to stop the itch/irritation in order to prevent further skin damage due to scratching.

Personally, I found pure aloe vera gel (from my plant) particularly soothing. Many of those online report using coconut oil with great benefit.

Soaking in a tub can relieve the itch/discomfort and prepare the skin for topicals. Finding any food triggers in your diet (sugar is a common instigator) can help reduce/eliminate itch. Including antihistamine foods into your diet may also assist (hence, the nettle tea).

Healing any abrasions, fissures or raw areas is the next goal.

There are a variety of healing salves on the market aimed directly at LS. It can get pricey, but it doesn't have to. Again, many report success using coconut oil, olive oil, or simple salves with natural ingredients.

If urine is aggravating, using a peri-bottle to rinse the vulva after peeing is an effective treatment for many with LS. One mom packed a special backpack for her daughter and educated the school nurse on her LS. Rather than deal with discomfort at school, her daughter could swing by the nurse's station on her way to the bathroom and grab her supplies. A post-pee rinse goes a long way to relieve discomfort and a topical application can further soothe the vulva. Smart mom.

Strengthen the skin barrier and protect the dermis.

As mentioned above, urine can irritate the skin. The peri-bottle or a bidet can work well to alleviate this. Some people find natural water wipes are better than toilet paper, especially when the skin is raw. As the skin heals, it needs protection. A barrier cream is useful, especially if underwear or pants cause friction (loose fitting clothing can help).

"Barrier creams maintain and protect the physical barrier of the skin and prevent the skin from drying out. They stop transepidermal water loss and skin breakdown by providing a topical barrier on the skin. These creams can also heal skin tears and existing wounds." By acting as a shield against potential irritants, they are designed to create the ideal environment for damaged skin to restore itself.[1]

ANNIE GONZALEZ, DERMATOLOGIST –
BYRDIE

Barrier creams tend to be thicker. Again, this can run the gamut of prices from the expensive blends to something as simple as castor oil. My PF therapist likes Cerave®. Emu oil is a popular choice in the LS community. While blends can offer a mixture of therapeutic ingredients, if one of the ingredients disagrees with your skin, it will be tricky to figure out the culprit.

Address the underlying inflammation.

We know that gut health plays a role in autoimmune conditions. It's important to improve the gut by reducing or eliminating processed foods, sugar and ingredients that cause sensitivity for you. You can have a naturopath test for these foods or keep a food journal to record any flares and what you've eaten. I've mentioned oxalates and histamines along with other dietary factors. I also covered oxidative stress and the vitamins and breathing practices that reduce OS. Include plenty of nutrient-dense foods in your diet.

Work to keep personal stress low and increase love and laughter in your life.

More Natural Avenues for Healing Lichen Sclerosus.

Again, LS is unique to each person. Some have reported good results using the following:

- Acupuncture and/or Traditional Chinese Medicine
- Homeopathy
- Mona Lisa Touch laser therapy
- PRP (platelet rich plasma injections)
- Naturopathy
- Functional medicine
- Herbology

And, of course, you'll find much information online:

Fractionated CO_2 laser treatment showed significant improvement in subjective symptoms and objective measures compared with clobetasol propionate, without serious safety or adverse events at 6 months.[2]

The National Library of Medicine's web page:

Topical and dietary administrations of avocado and soybean extract have been assessed in patients with mild to moderate vulvar lichen sclerosus (VLS). At the end of 24 weeks of treatment period, main sign and symptom of disease have been diminished significantly. **Conclusions:** Our results provide evidence that the topical and dietary supplements used in the study, which contain active principles exerting anti-inflammatory, anti-fibrotic, emollient, and lenitive actions, are effective alternatives in the treatment of symptoms and signs of mild-to-moderate VLS.[3]

It's up to you where you choose to invest your time, energy and money in your treatment plan. I've managed my LS well through diet, time in nature, meditation, rest, occasional soaks, vulvar tissue massage and daily topical oils/salves.

My current favourite blend of emollient that I make includes 5-6 drops of pomegranate seed oil from my health food store, a couple drops of vitamin E oil and a few drops of jojoba oil. This blend takes care of vitamins C, E and ceramides. It's lasted me months with good results.

Please note, that while I love a good mineral bath, I've not had the severity of fissures or rawness that others report. While soaking can be soothing, be mindful of using salts in the bath if you have open cuts. Some find it fine, while others find it painful. Start with a small amount and gradually increase if you go this route.

In the LS online groups, the word *cure* is avoided in favour of *remission*. Again, not a doctor. What most people with LS appear to be after is a routine that fosters remission and gives them the tools to personally manage any flares that crop up over time.

And, it goes without saying, this isn't meant to replace your doctor's advice or treatment. LS is a personal journey. You will find what works for you.

An LS Interview

I had the pleasure of interviewing Allicia Mae Cain, the administrator of the first LS Facebook group I joined. She is also the co-author of the book, *HELP! I Have Lichen Sclerosus! Hope for remission of LS symptoms via natural healing methods including Sodium tetraborate (borax) therapies.* I include the interview below for you.

What is the main issue you see in your Facebook group of members with LS?

A: Misdiagnosis and a lack of medical community who understand it.

Why did you create the group?

A: To get people talking about it (LS).

How long have you supported this group?

A: I had an original group I started in 2018 that got shut down. I reopened in early 2020 with a new name, thinking Facebook must not have liked something about the first name. There are over 5500 members, increasing every week.

What are you hoping will be the future of LS?

A: Educate more of the medical field. Personal awareness. Taking away some of the embarrassment and shame for those who are diagnosed with it.

If there was something you wished you'd known about LS when you wrote your book that you could add now, what would that be?

A: Pelvic floor therapy. I hadn't heard of it when we wrote our book.

What has helped you the most with your LS?

A: Originally the borax calmed my skin down from all the rawness, then the intermittent fasting became the best maintenance for me.

How long between your diagnosis and remission?

A: I received a diagnosis in 2010. I started in 2017 with internal healing (intermittent fasting). I'd say that in 2018 I was in remission.

What does remission mean to you?

A: You control the disease, the disease no longer controls you. I have the tools to remedy it.

You can find Allicia's Facebook group at Sharing is Caring About LS. [4]

The Power of Sangha

My children are with me every other week. This is the custody arrangement that created the healthiest scenario for our kids. During the week that they are not here, I schedule the majority of my appointments, work and can dive into my spiritual and health practices. Due to a change in schedule, the kids were with me for 10 days.

I noticed how challenging it was by the tenth day to manage my energy while assisting them with their needs. My son had Covid during that time and I kept my daughter home from school to keep things contained and everyone looked after. Honestly, I crushed it. That initial week went brilliantly. The following few days, however, were a shit show. We may love our families, however, we also need our sanghas.

A sangha is a community of friends practicing the dharma together in order to bring about and to maintain awareness. The essence of a sangha is awareness, understanding, acceptance, harmony and love. When you do not see these in a community, it is not a true sangha, and you should have the courage to say so.[5]

~*WHAT IS SANGHA* BY THICH NHAT HANH
IN LION'S ROAR MAGAZINE

Perhaps your family *is* your sangha. More times than not, though, I hear how people are striving to strike a balance between family and self-care. There's no right or wrong here. You can have your family and your sangha too.

When my beloved 22-year-old cat died last year, I was beside myself with grief. It was just before I discovered I had LS. I typically process these things alone, through writing, in nature or during meditation practice. At the time though, I was part of a year-long meditation commitment with a community of Tibetan Buddhist practitioners and students. I posted in our online community about my cat's death and my sadness. Of course, much love poured through the comments, however, one comment caught my attention and continues to float through my mind to this day. "The sangha is here for you."

I recognize that I am taking liberties with the term sangha here. In Thich Nhat Hanh's definition, he mentions a community practicing the *dharma*. Sangha is a Buddhist community. I also feel the same sense of sangha, however, in my qigong community. Why am I mentioning this? There is a difference between support groups and sangha:

The LS support groups have been invaluable in helping me to feel I'm not alone in this condition, offering information and resources. It's a place to share frustration, challenges and triumphs. It isn't a place I go for my personal healing practice.

What I'm saying is to consider finding your sangha. It may be a prayer group, your church or place of worship, qigong, Buddhism, meditation or yoga community. It might be a reiki share, Nia dance class, healing circle or even a gardening club. Make it a regular part of your wellness practice. Connect in person when possible. If that's not available, the world wide web is at your fingertips. Find a group that lifts your spirits and lightens your energy.

And yes, I'm pushing my personal agenda here.

1. Because I believe we are all connected, and that belonging to a loving community is not only good for the individual, it's good for the world.
2. Because you are so much more than your LS, and spiritual practice opens up the doors to a wider understanding of life, suffering and healing.
3. Because I want you to heal so that you can share even more love and healing energy with those around you.

Final Thoughts on LS

Be mindful not to exhaust your support people: friends and family. Having a conversation with your loved ones can help everyone set clear boundaries around what they are capable of giving. They already worry about your health. This is why it is important to find a support group where you can share the load. This allows your family, friends and partner to keep from being overwhelmed while also supporting you. Set up supports that nourish you *and* your relationships.

One of the members in the Facebook group questioned why LS seems to flare after diagnosis, that the condition seems to worsen after you've been told you have it. Two things come to mind here:

1. We are hypersensitive after diagnosis to anything happening in our vulvovaginal area. Before diagnosis, a minor itch would have gone scratched unnoticed, a little tingle and we simply recross our legs. Big itching and we take some cranberry juice or treat for yeast. After diagnosis, every itch becomes something to worry about.
2. Worry and anxiety. The reason I chose the subtitle for this book is that:

A. I don't want to mislead anyone into thinking I have the cure.

B. LS appears to have a strong correlation with stress and the very stress of dealing with and being diagnosed with LS can feel all-consuming.

We cannot know what life will bring, we can only fill our tool box with all the tools needed to nourish ourselves through our lifetime. If LS is where we are at this point in time, then let's use this opportunity to tend to our physical, mental and emotional wellbeing. Let's heal the stress of LS. And in that, we gain the tools to heal other stressors that may come our way.

I know it's hard to accept a gift that causes so much discomfort, pain, shame and often hopelessness. But people *are* healing from LS. Call it remission if you like, but people are healing. And LS is an opportunity to heal more than just our vulvas. As if that's not enough.

Do not compare your journey to another's. We each heal in our own time. And what if we don't heal? What of that? It can feel as though we failed somewhere. Not true, my friend. More formidable healers than you and me (and believe me, we are formidable) have yet to live in perfect health. Perhaps because that's not the point of life. We have never failed. We have always succeeded in living this precious human life.

So, do not take the weight of healing on your shoulders. Join the journey to nourish yourself in all ways. Choose self-compassion, kindness and light-heartedness when you can. When it's unbearable, offer it to Divine Mother, Mother Earth, your ancestors (I believe they had a role to play in this), and assemble your support team of physicians, pelvic floor specialists, family, friends, nature, your pets and your spiritual community or healing practices.

When Thich Nhat Hanh, the father of mindfulness and a beloved Buddhist teacher, died, I kept feeling this warmth as if he were still here for us all. While on my front step in gentle meditation, I felt him near and then felt the remarkable presence of Quan Yin, the *Bodhisattva* of compassion and a great healing goddess/saint.

When we practice compassion and loving kindness, we draw more of this energy for ourselves, our families, our communities and the world. How do you know you weren't tasked to take up this challenge? Offering compassion to your illness or pain draws more of this loving energy into the world. That's totally something I would have committed to.

I tend to take on big projects. I can see myself at the rebirth portal. "Yes, I'll sign up for two or three of those autoimmune thingies. That'll keep me committed to my practice and focused on healing the world."

Well, we don't have to heal the world. Just know that there is so much healing energy available to you. Enjoy finding a practice that warms your heart and ignites your spirit.

When I sat down to write this morning, I noticed I'd left a window open on my laptop that was supposed to broadcast a memorial practice for Thich Nhat Hanh. No memorial played. Instead, the Medicine Buddha Mantra rang out from Youtube. May its healing energy infuse these words and this book. May you find much support on your journey.

May you be happy
May you be healthy
May you be safe
May you be free from inner and outer suffering
May you live with ease and joy
And may all beings benefit.

MUCH LOVE,
Stephanie

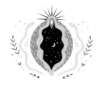

IF YOU ENJOYED THIS BOOK

Please leave a review on Amazon or your bookseller of choice. Your words help other readers to discover the book and support their journey to healing LS.

You also help Stephanie to continue doing the work she loves.

Thank you!

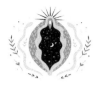

ABOUT THE AUTHOR

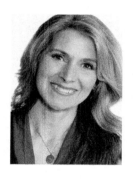

Stephanie Hrehirchuk is the author of 20 books, including the multi-award winning memoir, *An Accidental Awakening: It's not about yoga; It's about family.* Her passions and training over the years include Tibetan Breathing and Movement Yoga, raw nutrition, spinal reflexology, qigong, reiki and Ayurveda. Stephanie was diagnosed with LS in 2021 and shares her array of practices to support those with lichen sclerosus. Find her at StephanieHrehirchuk.com

ALSO BY STEPHANIE HREHIRCHUK

If you enjoyed the section on the chakras, pick up Stephanie's book:

Householder Yogini: Practices & Journaling Exercises for Women who Live at the Intersection of Spirituality & Family

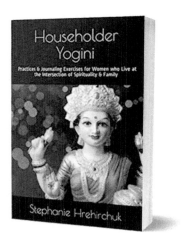

Stephanie includes a wealth of information, reflection questions, and examples for a healthy, peaceful, active way of being. She makes it feel easy to take action with a positive mindset. The exercises are helpful and practical. I highly recommend Householder Yogini.

JACQUIE C.

ALSO BY STEPHANIE HREHIRCHUK

Read Stephanie's multi award-winning memoir:

An Accidental Awakening: It's not about yoga; It's about family

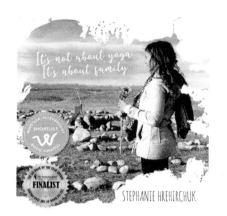

*Struggling to live with a young family, career,
and time for oneself is something most of us
relate to, and Stephanie tells it like it is and
opens our hearts to something rich and
rewarding as she plunges into her quest.*

CASSANDRA ARNOLD

ALSO BY STEPHANIE HREHIRCHUK

Create a nourishing daily ritual with:

Nourish: Ayurveda-inspired 21-day Detox

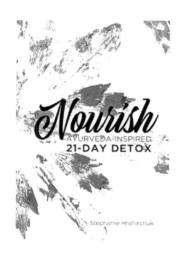

*The book is an easy read, geared towards real
people, with emphasis on nurturing your body.*

ER CAIRNS

ALSO BY STEPHANIE HREHIRCHUK

More books...

Awakening on Purpose: Trusting the call

Waking up the West: Return to Dreamtime

From Exercise to Ecstasy: 10 Ways to Turn Body-Mind into Body-Mind-Spirit

Children's Books

Anna and the Earth Angel

Anna and the Tree Fort

Anna and the Food Forest

Anna and the Christmas Tree

Grandfather Grasshopper

NOTES

Introduction

1. (Tysonsgynecology.com) Vulva-Vaginal Disorders Specialist & Vulva Dermatology - The Menopause Centre https://www.tysonsgynecology.com/vulva-dermatology-vaginal-disorders/
2. https://www.yourdictionary.com/vagina

1. The Lowdown on LS

1. Liberty Women's Health/ Vulvar Health: Lichen Sclerosus https://www.libertywomenshealth.ca/post/lichen-sclerosis
2. The Royal Women's Hospital, Victoria, Australia/ Lichen Sclerosus https://www.thewomens.org.au/health-information/vulva-vagina/vulva-vagina-problems/lichen-sclerosus
3. NORD/ Rare Disease Database/ Lichen Sclerosus https://rarediseases.org/rare-diseases/lichen-sclerosus/
4. National Human Genome Research Institute https://www.genome.gov/FAQ/Rare-Diseases#:
5. The Royal Women's Hospital, Victoria, Australia/ Lichen Sclerosus https://www.thewomens.org.au/health-information/vulva-vagina/vulva-vagina-problems/lichen-sclerosus
6. Tran DA, Tan X, Macri CJ, Goldstein AT, Fu SW. Lichen Sclerosus: An autoimmunopathogenic and genomic enigma with emerging genetic and immune targets. *Int J Biol Sci.* 2019;15(7):1429-1439. Published 2019 Jun 2. doi:10.7150/ijbs.34613
7. (Healthline.com) Corinne O'Keefe Osborn, January, 2019 https://www.healthline.com/health/lichenification#:
8. https://www.merriam-webster.com/dictionary/sclerosis#:~:text=1%20%3A%20pathological%20hardening%20of%20tissue,adapt%20or%20compromise%20political%20sclerosis
9. https://www.youtube.com/watch?v=vltY9mr8E68
10. Fistarol SK, Itin PH. Diagnosis and treatment of lichen sclerosus: an update. *Am J Clin Dermatol.* 2013;14(1):27-47. doi:10.1007/s40257-012-0006-4
11. (ClinicalAdvisor.com) Melissa Morgan & Lisa Daitch, February, 2017 https://www.clinicaladvisor.com/home/topics/ob-gyn-information-center/vulvar-lichen-sclerosus-breaking-the-silence/

12. (CedarsSinai.com) Lichen Sclerosus https://www.cedars-sinai.org/health-library/diseases-and-conditions/l/lichen-sclerosus.html

13. The Royal Children's Hospital Melbourne, July 2020 https://www.rch.org.au/kidsinfo/fact_sheets/Lichen_sclerosus/

14. (MountainRoseHerbs.com) Borax Powder https://mountainroseherbs.com/borax-powder

15. (Healthline.com) Erica Cerino, May, 2018 https://www.healthline.com/health/is-borax-safe

2. The Road to Healing

1. (Today.com) Kamari Stewart, November, 2021 https://www.today.com/shop/ceramides-benefits-products-t237467

2. (Healthline.com) Kristeen Cherney, August, 2018 https://www.healthline.com/health/beauty-skin-care/ceramide#takeaway

3. (my.clevelandclinic.org) Lichen Sclerosus https://my.clevelandclinic.org/health/diseases/16564-lichen-sclerosus

4. (thelancet.com) Dr. JJ Powell & F Wojnarowska, May, 1999 https://www.thelancet.com/journals/lancet/article/PIIS0140-6736(98)08228-2/references

5. Nilanchali Singh, Prafull Ghatage, "Etiology, Clinical Features, and Diagnosis of Vulvar Lichen Sclerosus: A Scoping Review", *Obstetrics and Gynecology International*, vol. 2020, Article ID 7480754, 8 pages, 2020. https://doi.org/10.1155/2020/7480754

6. Kirtschig G. Lichen Sclerosus-Presentation, Diagnosis and Management. *Dtsch Arztebl Int.* 2016;113(19):337-343. doi:10.3238/arztebl.2016.0337 https://www.ncbi.nlm.nih.gov/pmc/articles/PMC4904529/

7. (Humanwindow.com) Martin Caparrotta, September, 2020 https://humanwindow.com/dr-gabor-mate-interview-childhood-trauma-anxiety-culture/

8. (BBC.com) Claudia Hammond, Can Writing About Pain Make You Heal Faster, June, 2017 https://www.bbc.com/future/article/20170601-can-writing-about-pain-make-you-heal-faster

9. (my.Clevelandclinic.org) Stress https://my.clevelandclinic.org/health/articles/11874-stress

10. (Drgabormate.com) Home https://drgabormate.com/mindbody-health/

11. Paulis G, Berardesca E. Lichen sclerosus: the role of oxidative stress in the pathogenesis of the disease and its possible transformation into carcinoma. *Res Rep Urol.* 2019;11:223-232. Published 2019 Aug 20. doi:10.2147/RRU.S205184 https://www.ncbi.nlm.nih.gov/pmc/articles/PMC6709801/

12. Serbecic N, Beutelspacher SC. Anti-oxidative vitamins prevent lipid-peroxidation and apoptosis in corneal endothelial cells. *Cell Tissue Res.* 2005;320(3):465-475. doi:10.1007/s00441-004-1030-3

https://pubmed.ncbi.nlm.nih.gov/15838641/

13. Lee CH, Giuliani F. The Role of Inflammation in Depression and Fatigue. *Front Immunol.* 2019;10:1696. Published 2019 Jul 19. doi:10.3389/fimmu.2019.01696 https://www.ncbi.nlm.nih.gov/pmc/articles/PMC6658985/

14. Martarelli D, Cocchioni M, Scuri S, Pompei P. Diaphragmatic breathing reduces exercise-induced oxidative stress. *Evid Based Complement Alternat Med.* 2011;2011:932430. doi:10.1093/ecam/nep169 https://www.ncbi.nlm.nih.gov/pmc/articles/PMC3139518/

15. Yang, E.J., Sekhon, S., Beck, K.M. *et al.* Neuromodulation in Inflammatory Skin Disease. *Dermatol Ther (Heidelb)* **8,** 1–4 (2018). https://doi.org/10.1007/s13555-018-0227-4 https://link.springer.com/article/10.1007/s13555-018-0227-4

16. (CBC.ca) Nicole Mahabir, From fight or flight to rest and digest: How to reset your nervous system with breath, January, 2018
https://www.cbc.ca/life/wellness/from-fight-or-flight-to-rest-and-digest-how-to-reset-your-nervous-system-with-the-breath-1.4485695

17. (hopkinsallchildrens.org) Diaphragmatic Breathing https://www.hopkinsallchildrens.org/Services/Anesthesiology/Pain-Management/Complementary-Pain-Therapies/Diaphragmatic-Breathing

18. (Physiotherapy.ca) Samantha Doralp, Spotlight on Alternative Nostril Breathing https://physiotherapy.ca/spotlight-alternate-nostril-breathing

3. From Food to Fasting

1. (Hopkinsmedicine.org) Intermittent Fasting: What is it, and how does it work? https://www.hopkinsmedicine.org/health/wellness-and-prevention/intermittent-fasting-what-is-it-and-how-does-it-work

2. (Cedars-sinai.org) Agata Smieciuszewski, Is Intermittent Fasting Healthy? November, 2019 https://www.cedars-sinai.org/blog/intermittent-fasting.html

3. (Sydneygastroenterologist.com.au) How too much sugar affects the gut microbiome http://sydneygastroenterologist.com.au/blog/how-too-much-sugar-affects-the-gut-microbiome/

4. Chattopadhyay S, Arnold JD, Malayil L, et al. Potential role of the skin and gut microbiota in premenarchal vulvar lichen sclerosus: A pilot case-control study. *PLoS One.* 2021;16(1):e0245243. Published 2021 Jan 14. doi:10.1371/journal.pone.0245243 https://pubmed.ncbi.nlm.nih.gov/33444404/

5. (Glutenfreesociety.org) Research Links Gluten Sensitivity to Multiple Autoimmune Diseases https://www.glutenfreesociety.org/gluten-and-the-autoimmune-disease-spectrum/

6. (Urologyofva.net) The Damaging Effects of Oxalates on the Human Body https://www.urologyofva.net/articles/category/healthy-living/3740469/11/13/2019/the-damaging-effects-of-oxalates-on-the-human-body

7. (Blog.rhealthc.com) Rebecca Maas, What You Need to Know about the Oxalates in Your Diet, April, 2021 https://blog.rhealthc.com/what-you-need-to-know-about-the-oxalates-in-your-diet/

8. (Sallynorton.com) Sally K Norton, What is oxalate and how can it impact your health? https://sallyknorton.com/oxalate-science/oxalate-basics/

9. (Vulvalpainsociety.org) TREATMENT OF VULVODYNIA https://vulvalpainsociety.org/research/published-research/#Holistic

10. (Hoffmancentre.com) Bruce Hoffman, Are High Oxalate Levels Harming Your Health?, August, 2021 https://hoffmancentre.com/are-high-oxalate-levels-harming-your-health/

11. (Drbeckycampbell.com) Dr. Becky Campbell, The Histamine and Blood Sugar Connection https://drbeckycampbell.com/histamine-blood-sugar-connection/

12. Farrell AM, Millard PR, Schomberg KH, Wojnarowska F. An infective aetiology for vulval lichen sclerosus re-addressed. *Clin Exp Dermatol.* 1999;24(6):479-483. doi:10.1046/j.1365-2230.1999.00538.x https://pubmed.ncbi.nlm.nih.gov/10606954/

13. (Healinghistamine.com) Histamine Intolerance, Mast Cells & Autoimmune Disorders https://healinghistamine.com/blog/histamine-mast-cells-autoimmune-disorders/

14. (Drruscio.com) Dr. Michael Ruscio, Causes of Histamine Intolerance and How to Overcome It, November, 2020 https://drruscio.com/everything-you-need-to-know-about-histamine-intolerance/

15. Chung BY, Park SY, Byun YS, et al. Effect of Different Cooking Methods on Histamine Levels in Selected Foods. *Ann Dermatol.* 2017;29(6):706-714. doi:10.5021/ad.2017.29.6.706 https://www.ncbi.nlm.nih.gov/pmc/articles/PMC5705351/

16. (lanisimpson.com) Nettles for Bones and More! May, 2010 https://lanisimpson.com/blogs/news/nettles-for-bones-and-more

17. Kregiel D, Pawlikowska E, Antolak H. *Urtica* spp.: Ordinary Plants with Extraordinary Properties. *Molecules.* 2018;23(7):1664. Published 2018 Jul 9. doi:10.3390/molecules23071664 https://www.ncbi.nlm.nih.gov/pmc/articles/PMC6100552/

18. (Healthline.com) Ryan Raman, November, 2018, 6 Evidence-based Benefits of Stinging Nettle https://www.healthline.com/nutrition/stinging-nettle#TOC_TITLE_HDR_9

4. Supporting the Vulva

1. Günthert AR, Limacher A, Beltraminelli H, et al. Efficacy of topical progesterone versus topical clobetasol propionate in patients with vulvar Lichen sclerosus - A double-blind randomized phase II pilot study. *Eur J Obstet Gynecol Reprod Biol.* 2022;272:88-95. doi:10.1016/j.ejogrb.2022.03.020 https://pubmed.ncbi.nlm.nih.gov/35290878/

2. Goldman RD. Child health update: estrogen cream for labial adhesion in girls. *Can Fam Physician*. 2013;59(1):37-38. https://www.ncbi.nlm.nih.gov/pmc/articles/PMC3555651/

3. (Health.harvard.edu) Celeste Robb-Nicholson, By the way, doctor: Is vaginal estrogen safe? August, 2021
    https://www.health.harvard.edu/womens-health/by-the-way-doctor-is-vaginal-estrogen-safe

4. (Cancertherapyadvisor.com) Lori Boardman, Vulvovaginal Disorders: Lichen Sclerosus https://www.cancertherapyadvisor.com/home/decision-support-in-medicine/obstetrics-and-gynecology/vulvovaginal-disorders-lichen-sclerosus/

5. Renaud-Vilmer C, Cavelier-Balloy B, Porcher R, Dubertret L. Vulvar Lichen Sclerosus: Effect of Long-term Topical Application of a Potent Steroid on the Course of the Disease. *Arch Dermatol*. 2004;140(6):709–712.   doi:10.1001/archderm.140.6.709   https://jamanetwork.com/journals/jamadermatology/fullarticle/480623

6. Lee A, Bradford J, Fischer G. Long-term Management of Adult Vulvar Lichen Sclerosus: A Prospective Cohort Study of 507 Women. *JAMA Dermatol*.   2015;151(10):1061-1067. doi:10.1001/jamadermatol.2015.0643
    https://pubmed.ncbi.nlm.nih.gov/26070005/

7. Nilanchali Singh, Neha Mishra, Prafull Ghatage, Treatment Options in Vulvar Lichen Sclerosus: A Scoping Review, February, 2021 https://www.cureus.com/articles/49721-treatment-options-in-vulvar-lichen-sclerosus-a-scoping-review

8. (Cancer.org) Survival Rates for Vulvar Cancer https://www.cancer.org/cancer/vulvar-cancer/detection-diagnosis-staging/survival-rates.html

9. (Mayoclinic.org) Vaginal Atrophy https://www.mayoclinic.org/diseases-conditions/vaginal-atrophy/symptoms-causes/syc-20352288

10. (Racgp.org.au) Elizabeth Farrell, Genitourinary syndrome of menopause, July, 2017 https://www.racgp.org.au/afp/2017/july/genitourinary-syndrome-of-menopause

5. An Alternative Approach

1. (Tysonsgynecology.com) Adrenal Fatigue and Menopause https://www.tysonsgynecology.com/adrenal-fatigue-and-menopause/

2. (Health.Harvard.edu) Giving Thanks Can Make You Happier, August, 2021   https://www.health.harvard.edu/healthbeat/giving-thanks-can-make-you-happier

3. (Greatergood.berkeley.edu) Joshua Brown & Joel Wong| How Gratitude Changes You and Your Brain, June 6, 2017 https://greatergood.berkeley.edu/article/item/how_gratitude_changes_you_and_your_brain

4. (Autoimmuneinstitute.org) Margaux Thieme-Burdette, What is Gratitude, November 10, 2021 https://www.autoimmuneinstitute.org/what-is-gratitude/

5. (Sciencedaily.com) Cincinnati Children's Hospital Medical Centre, 'Mono' virus linked to seven serious diseases, April, 2018 https://www.sciencedaily.com/releases/2018/04/180416121606.htm

6. (Mayoclinic.org) Mayo Clinic staff, Meditation: A simple, fast way to reduce stress https://www.mayoclinic.org/tests-procedures/meditation/in-depth/meditation/art-20045858

7. (Newscientist.com) Joe Marchant, June, 2017, Mindfulness and meditation dampen down inflammation genes
    https://www.newscientist.com/article/2137595-mindfulness-and-meditation-dampen-down-inflammation-genes/#ixzz7RUy4y7eR

8. (Theacupunctureclinic.co.nz) Heiko Lade, Chinese Herbs For Lichen Sclerosus, September, 2017 https://www.theacupunctureclinic.co.nz/chinese-herbs-for-lichen-sclerosus/

6. A Nourishing Ritual

1. (Byrdie.com) Amy Lewis, How to Use Barrier Creams (and the 10 Best Ones to Use), March, 2022 https://www.byrdie.com/what-are-barrier-creams

2. (Nva.org) Linda S. Burkett, MD, Moiuri Siddique, MD, MPH, Alexander Zeymo, MS, Elizabeth A. Brunn, MD, Robert E. Gutman, MD, Amy J. Park, MD, and Cheryl B. Iglesia, MD/ From the Department of Obstetrics and Gynecology/ Clobetasol Compared With Fractionated Carbon Dioxide Laser for Lichen Sclerosus, June, 2021 https://www.nva.org/wp-content/uploads/2021/09/Clobetasol-Compared-With-Fractionated.pdf

3. Ghasemian M, Owlia S, Owlia MB. Review of Anti-Inflammatory Herbal Medicines. *Adv Pharmacol Sci.* 2016;2016:9130979. doi:10.1155/2016/9130979 https://www.ncbi.nlm.nih.gov/pmc/articles/PMC4877453/

4. Sharing is caring about LS https://www.facebook.com/groups/1329440753906331/

5.)Lionsroar.com) Thich Nhat Hanh/ What Is Sangha?/ *Friends on the Path: Living Spiritual Communities* (2002) https://www.lionsroar.com/the-practice-of-sangha/

Printed in Great Britain
by Amazon

34882022R00088

in 11+ tests

11+
English
Success

| Age 6–7 |
| Age 7–8 |
| **Age 8–9** |
| Age 9–10 |
| Age 10–11 |

Assessment Papers

Alison Head

Sample page

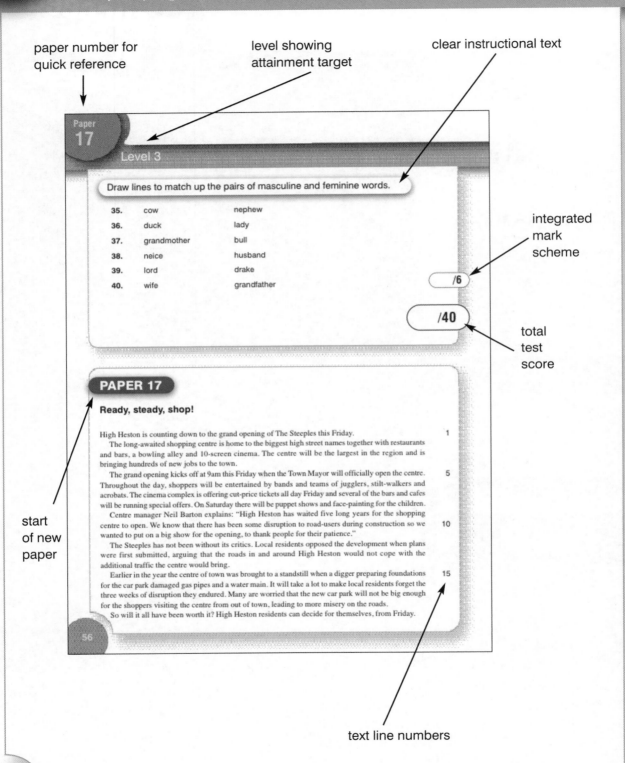

paper number for quick reference

level showing attainment target

clear instructional text

Paper 17

Level 3

Draw lines to match up the pairs of masculine and feminine words.

35. cow — nephew
36. duck — lady
37. grandmother — bull
38. neice — husband
39. lord — drake
40. wife — grandfather

integrated mark scheme

/6

/40

total test score

PAPER 17

start of new paper

Ready, steady, shop!

High Heston is counting down to the grand opening of The Steeples this Friday.　1
　　The long-awaited shopping centre is home to the biggest high street names together with restaurants and bars, a bowling alley and 10-screen cinema. The centre will be the largest in the region and is bringing hundreds of new jobs to the town.
　　The grand opening kicks off at 9am this Friday when the Town Mayor will officially open the centre.　5
Throughout the day, shoppers will be entertained by bands and teams of jugglers, stilt-walkers and acrobats. The cinema complex is offering cut-price tickets all day Friday and several of the bars and cafes will be running special offers. On Saturday there will be puppet shows and face-painting for the children.
　　Centre manager Neil Barton explains: "High Heston has waited five long years for the shopping centre to open. We know that there has been some disruption to road-users during construction so we　10
wanted to put on a big show for the opening, to thank people for their patience."
　　The Steeples has not been without its critics. Local residents opposed the development when plans were first submitted, arguing that the roads in and around High Heston would not cope with the additional traffic the centre would bring.
　　Earlier in the year the centre of town was brought to a standstill when a digger preparing foundations　15
for the car park damaged gas pipes and a water main. It will take a lot to make local residents forget the three weeks of disruption they endured. Many are worried that the new car park will not be big enough for the shoppers visiting the centre from out of town, leading to more misery on the roads.
　　So will it all have been worth it? High Heston residents can decide for themselves, from Friday.

56

text line numbers

2

Contents

PAPER 1

It had been a thoroughly ordinary Thursday. Assembly in the hall was followed by a maths test. Playtime was inside because of the rain, then PE and art, which was making firework pictures on black paper with coloured chalks. Cheese spread sandwiches for lunch, then more wet play. English came after lunch, writing stories about the autumn.

It was strange, then, that the walk home from school should turn out to be quite so extraordinary. As usual, Joe walked with his friend Max as far as the corner, before saying goodbye and heading for home in the next street.

"Excuse me," said a voice, politely. "I appear to be a bit stuck." Joe looked up and down the empty street. He thought he must be hearing things. After all, what would you think if you heard someone speaking to you when there was nobody there?

"Please don't walk past!" begged the voice. Listening carefully, Joe followed the sound of the voice across the pavement. It seemed to be coming from… Joe peered down the drain and found himself gazing into a pair of large, scared eyes. He gasped.

Circle the correct answers.

1. What was Joe's first lesson after assembly?

English   maths   art

2. What was in Joe's sandwiches?

jam   ham   cheese spread

3. What was Joe's friend called?

Martin   Mark   Max

Answer these questions.

4. How did Joe make his firework picture?

_____

_____

5. What was the weather like in the story?

_____

6–7. The story takes place in the autumn. Write down two things in the story that tell you that.

_____

_____

8. Explain in your own words how you would feel if you heard a voice speaking to you when there was nobody there.

_____

_____

_____

_____

9. What do you think the word *gasped* means in the final line of the text?

_____

_____

_____

10. Why do you think Joe gasped when he saw a pair of eyes looking at him from the drain?

_____

_____

/10

Underline an **adjective** in each line.

11.	book	speak	green	buy
12.	happy	farm	give	school
13.	Sunday	beach	huge	ear
14.	dark	journey	friend	prettily
15.	tea	build	under	frosty
16.	shoe	dog	soft	box

/6

Write down a *le* word for each picture.

17. candle

18. table

19. cradle

20. bottle

21. stable

22. ankle

/6

Add the prefix *un* or *dis* to make antonyms.

23. un happy

24. dis qualify

25. dis appear

26. un fair

27. un pack

28. dis agree

/6

Write down the separate words that make up these **compound words**.

29–30. doorbell _____door_____ _____bell_____

31–32. cheesecake _____cheese_____ _____cake_____

33–34. earring _____ear_____ _____ring_____

/6

Write these words again, in **alphabetical order**.

green orange pink blue purple red

35. _____   36. _____

37. _____   38. _____

39. _____   40. _____

/6

/40

PAPER 2

The Sahara Desert

The Sahara is the world's largest hot desert. It covers more than nine million square miles,   1
making it larger than Australia and almost as big as Europe.

The desert covers vast areas of North Africa including large parts of Egypt, Libya, Tunisia,
Chad and Morocco. It was once a much wetter place than it is today, and fossils show
that dinosaurs once lived there. Today, most of the Sahara is covered with rocks and   5
sand dunes, which can reach 180 metres high.

Two and a half million people live in the Sahara Desert, mostly in Egypt, Algeria, Tunisia
and Morocco. Out of the cities, people use dromedary camels to get about. They are
specially adapted for life in the desert, with large, flat feet for walking on the sand
and long eyelashes to keep sand grains out of their eyes. They use their fatty humps to   10
store water, enabling them to stay in the desert for long periods of time. Their thick coats
help to keep them warm when the temperatures drop sharply at night.

Few plants grow in the desert apart from in the fertile Nile valley and in oases, which are
lakes made by natural spring water. The Nile is the world's longest river and Egypt's people
have relied on its waters for survival for thousands of years. The ancient Egyptian   15
civilisation grew up along its banks and the remains of countless temples and pyramids
can still be seen today, preserved by the hot, dry desert air.

Circle the correct answers.

1. The Sahara Desert is almost as large as which continent?

Europe   Asia   America

2. Plants grow in oases in the desert. Why do you think this is?

because oases have water   because oases are dry   because oases have sand

Answer these questions.

3–5. List three countries covered by the Sahara Desert.

Libia   _Morocco_   _egypt_

6. How do we know that dinosaurs once lived there?

fossils

7. What does the word *dune* mean in line 6?

Pile of sand that can reach 15 metres high

8–9. Write down two ways that camels are adapted for life in the desert.

humps with water flat feet for walking in sand.

10. Explain in your own words why an animal that lives in the desert might need a thick coat.

at night it's cold

/10

Underline the **homonym** in each pair.

11.	saw gate	**12.**	room right
13.	learn tap	**14.**	ball flower
15.	train rug	**16.**	light pen

/6

Write down the **plural** form of these **singular nouns**.

17. ~~egg~~   eggs

18. ~~fish~~

19. ~~glove~~

20. ~~witch~~   witches

21. ~~bus~~

22. ~~zoo~~   boxes

/6

Underline the **verb** in each sentence.

23. The girl climbed the stairs.

24. Flowers grow in the park.

25. A flock of birds flew over our garden.

26. My brother plays basketball for his school.

27. The cat balanced on the fence.

28. Sarah wandered slowly to school.

/6

Circle the words that have two **syllables**.

29–34.   hospital   pillow   rabbit   house

follow   beach   candle   computer

coach   fortune   bubble

/6

Add the **suffix** *ful* or *ly* to each of these words.

35.   kind_____   36.   hope_____

37.   forget_____   38.   actual_____

39.   like_____   40.   pain_____

/6

/40

PAPER 3

New Home for Newtown School

Councillors have blown the whistle on a school's plans for expansion with the announcement this   1
week that Newtown School will close at the end of the school year.

Head teacher Robin Shaw approached the council last year looking for funding to extend the
school buildings, which are no longer large enough to accommodate the school's 240 pupils.
Reviewing the application, the council has decided that the upkeep of the site, constructed in 1950,   5
has become too costly. It has purchased a site across town where a new school is planned. The current
Newtown site will be sold for housing development.

The decision has angered parents, who worry about the long and difficult journey their children
will face to get to school each day. Sally Groves, mother of eight-year-old Emily says, "It will take
Emily more than half an hour to walk to school and she will have to cross three major roads to get   10
there. If parents have to drive to the school, we'll just be adding to the rush-hour traffic. The council
hasn't thought this through."

Town Councillor Jenny Green disagrees. "As a council we have to make decisions about the best
way to spend taxpayers' money. Newtown School was constructed after the war with reinforced
concrete, which is now crumbling. It would not be practical to extend the existing buildings. The new   15
school will have fantastic facilities and enjoy better transport links, with a frequent bus service and
new pedestrian crossings. There will also be traffic-calming measures in the local area, including
speed bumps, to slow the traffic down.

Selling off the Newtown site to Harris Homes would also provide the council with a significant
source of income, enabling us to improve services to local residents. It is a win-win situation."   20

Local residents have until the end of next week to oppose the plan.

Circle the correct answers.

1. Why did the head teacher want funding?

    to build a new school   to extend the school   to pay for a school trip

2. Why was this?

    the buildings were   the buildings   the buildings were not
       crumbling   were old   big enough

Answer these questions.

3–4. Write down two reasons Sally Groves is worried about her daughter walking to the new
school.

_____

_____

5. Why does Jenny Green say that the existing school buildings could not be extended?

_____

_____

6–7. Explain in your own words two effects that the location of the new school might have on local roads.

_____

_____

_____

8. Give an example of a *traffic-calming measure* (line 17) that is mentioned in the text.

_____

9. Who wants to buy the old Newtown School site?

_____

10. What does Councillor Green mean when she describes the construction of the new school as a "win-win situation"?

_____

_____

/10

Add *there* or *their* to complete each sentence.

11. We will go sledging if _____ is snow.

12. _____ will be time to play after tea.

13. The boys left _____ muddy shoes by the door.

14. I love the park so we go _____ every Sunday.

15. The horses flick _____ tails to brush away the flies.

16. The actors learnt _____ lines for the school play.

/6

Write down an **antonym** for each word.

17. high _____

18. big _____

19. lost _____

20. empty _____

21. clean _____

22. tall _____

/6

Write these **present tense** sentences again, in the **past tense**.

23. Ben walks to school. _____

24. The girls collect shells on the beach. _____

25. I wish by the wishing well. _____

26. Mum bakes cherry cakes. _____

27. I switch on the lights at night time. _____

28. Sally brushes her long hair. _____

/6

Circle the correctly spelt word in each pair.

29. table   tabble

30. buble   bubble

31. carry   cary

32. happy   hapy

33. peper   pepper

34. summer   sumer

/6

Write down the words that have been joined in each **contraction**.

35. I'm _____

36. she'll _____

37. couldn't _____

38. they're _____

39. he's _____

40. we'll _____

/6

/40

PAPER 4

Gingerbread men

Ginger is a natural flavouring made from the root of a plant. It is delicious in biscuits and cakes and is also used in Eastern cookery.

To make 16 gingerbread men you will need:

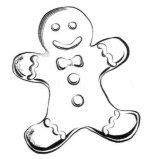

Ingredients
- 200g plain flour
- Pinch of salt
- 1 x 10ml spoon of ground ginger
- 75g butter or margarine
- 50g sugar
- 75g golden syrup

cutter
- 2 eggs
- Currants for decoration
- Flour for rolling out
- Butter for greasing the baking sheet

Equipment
- Weighing scales
- Mixing bowl
- Wooden spoon
- Rolling pin
- Baking sheet
- Gingerbread man

1. Heat the oven to 180° Celsius.
2. Thoroughly mix together the butter, sugar and syrup.
3. Add the flour, ginger and salt.
4. Beat the egg and add enough to the mixture to make a stiff dough.
5. Dust your work surface with flour to prevent the dough from sticking.
6. Use a rolling pin to roll out the dough half a centimetre thick.
7. Cut out gingerbread men with a cutter.
8. Add currants for eyes, noses, mouths and buttons.
9. Bake on a greased baking sheet for 20 minutes.
10. Allow to cool on a cooling rack before storing in an airtight container.

Circle the correct answers.

1. What kind of flour is used in the recipe?

    self-raising   wholemeal   plain

2. What should you use to prevent the mixture from sticking to the work surface?

    dust   flour   sugar

3. What are the currants for?

    decoration   flavour   rolling out

Answer these questions.

4. What is a *natural flavouring?*

_____

_____

5. Explain in your own words what the phrase *pinch of salt* means.

_____

_____

6. Why do you think the syrup has the name *golden syrup*?

_____

_____

7. Why should you grease the baking sheet with butter?

_____

_____

Write down what these words in the recipe mean.

8. Ingredients _____

9. Equipment _____

10. Air-tight container _____ /10

Find the **proper nouns** then write them again with capital letters.

bag	swan	france	dog	october
monday	door	window	sally	liam
cushion	europe	lamp		

11. _____ **12.** _____ **13.** _____

14. _____ **15.** _____ **16.** _____ /6

Choose *am*, *is* or *are* to complete each sentence.

17. I _____ going to Spain on holiday.

18. My dog _____ called Wendy.

19. I can join the judo club when I _____ nine.

20. I like my cousins because they _____ great fun.

21. Owls _____ nocturnal animals.

22. It _____ cold today.

/6

Underline the **personal pronoun** in each sentence.

23. We were late because the alarm clock was broken.

24. Dad was delighted because he won the football match.

25. Mum made us pizza for tea.

26. I would love to go rock climbing.

27. You must cross the road carefully.

28. Mum and Dad are grumpy when they wake up in the morning.

/6

Circle a **synonym** for each of these words.

29. **old**	broken	ancient	short
30. **ocean**	sea	lake	watch
31. **worried**	cheerful	concerned	delighted
32. **road**	church	school	street
33. **answer**	question	reply	suggest
34. **house**	shed	home	sock

/6

Underline the **root word** inside each longer word.

35. export   **36.** hopeful   **37.** heroic

38. winner   **39.** golden   **40.** realistic   /6

/40

PAPER 5

Weird is the woman who lives in the woods   1
and weird are the clothes she wears.
Crooked the roof of her gingerbread house
and crooked the rickety stairs.
Tattered and patched are the curtains that hide   5
the tattered and patched things decaying inside.

Sneaky and cheeky the children who spy,
leaving their safe little homes nearby.
Creaky and squeaky footsteps on the floor,
creaky and squeaky the hinge on the door.   10
No time to run from what stands there…
a tiny old lady with bugs in her hair.

"Come in my dears, I'm about to have dinner.
I'll disappear if I get any thinner!
I look forward to children coming to snoop,   15
it gives me something to put in my soup!"

Circle the phrase to correct this question.

1. What kind of stories do gingerbread houses sometimes appear in? Circle your answer.

crime stories   fairytales   science fiction stories

Answer these questions.

2–3. Write down two words that describe the stairs.

_____   _____

4. What does the word *decaying* mean in line 6?

_____

5. Why do you think the children come to spy?

_____

6–7. Write down two words in the second verse that describe sounds coming from inside the house.

_____   _____

8. What is unusual about the old lady's hair?

_____

9. What does the lady say she was about to do?

_____

10. What does she want to put in her soup?

_____   /10

11–16. Write these words again in **alphabetical order**.

come grape soil camel sausage giant

1 _____   2 _____   3 _____

4 _____   5 _____   6 _____   /6

Pick a sequencing word from the box to fill each gap.

After, then, Next, First, before, finally

17–22. _____, Grandad filled little pots with compost, _____ using a pencil to make a little hole in the soil. _____, he dropped a seed into each hole, _____ he gently covered the seed with compost. _____ that he watered each pot carefully and _____ he placed them on the windowsill in the sunlight.

/6

Add the **suffix** *ship* or *hood* to these words.

23. child_____

24. knight_____

25. friend_____

26. boy_____

27. owner_____

28. neighbour_____

29. partner_____

30. member_____

/8

In each sentence, underline the words that someone has said.

31. "What a beautiful picture!" said the teacher.

32. Dad called up the stairs, "Have you seen my keys?"

33. Poppy shouted, "Great goal!"

34. "We'll be late if we don't hurry!" warned Mum.

/4

Add the **possessive apostrophe** in the correct place.

35. the dogs paw

36. the womans car

37. a cats tail

38. the girls foot

39. a towns roads

40. the boys nose

/6

/40

PAPER 6

The Heart of the Monkey
(based on an African Swahili folk tale)

A long time ago, a little town stood at the foot of a cliff. On the edge
of the town grew an enormous kuyu tree. It was so large that half of
its branches grew over the town and the other half grew out over the sea.

1

The branches of the tree were heavy with fruit and a large grey monkey sat in the tree
each morning to eat his breakfast. One day he noticed a shark watching him greedily.

5

"Oh, if only I could have some of that fruit. I am so tired of salty fish," complained
the shark.

The monkey threw down some kuyu fruit and from that day the monkey and the shark ate
breakfast together each morning. One day, the monkey said, "How I wish I could see all
the wonderful things in the sea."

10

The crafty shark replied, "Hop on my back and I will show you those things. I promise that
you won't even get wet."

The monkey agreed, and the pair set off together on a long journey. Six days later the shark
said, "I have something to tell you, monkey. Before we left on our journey, I heard that
the sultan of my country is terribly ill and can only be cured with the heart of a monkey."

15

The frightened monkey thought carefully, then replied. "What a pity you did not tell me
when I was still on land. Then I would have brought my heart with me."

"Whatever do you mean?" asked the puzzled shark.

"Surely you must know that when we go on a journey we leave our hearts hanging in a
tree, so that they will not trouble us?"

20

The disappointed shark said, "There is no point going on if you
don't have your heart. We had better go back for it."

The monkey was delighted, but careful not to show it. The shark swam quickly and within
three days they were back at the kuyu tree. The monkey swung himself into the tree. As
he disappeared into the branches he called, "Have a pleasant journey home. I hope you
find your sultan better!"

25

1. What sat in the tree to eat its breakfast? Circle your answer.

    a parrot   a monkey   a squirrel

2. Find and write down one word in the first paragraph that comes from another language.

_____

3. What reason does the shark give for wanting some fruit?

_____

4–5. Find and write down two words used to describe the shark in the story.

_____   _____

6. What does the word *sultan* (line 15) mean?

_____

_____

7. Why is the monkey afraid in line 16?

_____

_____

8. Explain in your own words how the monkey tricks the shark into taking him back home.

_____

_____

9. How long, altogether, were the monkey and the shark travelling?

_____

10. Write a sentence to explain which of the animals in the story you think is wiser.
Include evidence from the story.

_____

_____   /10

Add a **comma** to each sentence to mark where the reader should pause.

11. Anna wrote as neatly as she could not smudging the ink at all.

12. Tail wagging wildly the puppy chased the ball.

13. Not finding any boots she liked Nina bought some shoes instead.

14. When nobody answered the phone Max left a message.   /4

Add *ly* to these words to turn them into **adverbs**.
Remember to alter the spelling if necessary.

15. kind _____

16. pretty_____

17. actual _____

18. dainty_____

19. full _____

20. dizzy_____

21. rude _____

22. graceful_____

/8

Read this passage, then answer the questions.

The children of Jubilee Road all play together. Eight year-old Paulo lives at number 2, next to Laura who is nearly 10 and her older brother Mark, who is 12. Three doors down live twins Daniel and Christopher, who are nine. When it snows they all go sledging together and in the summer holidays they like to camp out in their back gardens. Whatever they do, Mark is normally in charge.

23. Who is the oldest child in Jubilee Road?

_____

24. How many of the children are nine years old?

_____

25. Who has no brothers or sisters?

_____

26. Suggest a reason why Mark normally takes charge of the group.

_____

/4

Circle the correct **diminutive** for each bold word.

27. pig   pigling   piglet

28. duck   ducklet   duckling

29. goose gosling   gooselet

30. cat   catkin   kitten

31. swan   cygnet   swanlet

32. horse   calf   foal

33. bear   cub   pup

34. kangaroo roo   joey

/8

Use one of the **conjunctions** from the box to complete each sentence.

> when   because   before   but   so   while

35. We waited at our friend's house _____ Mum was finishing her work.

36. It was very funny _____ Dad fell over on the ice.

37. My sister won the prize _____ her entry was the best.

38. We bought the best tickets for the show _____ we would have the best view.

39. We ran to catch the bus _____ we were too late.

40. Dad made us breakfast _____ he left for work.

/6

/40

PAPER 7

Swanage, Dorset
A visitor's guide

The seaside town of Swanage lies at the end of the Purbeck peninsula. Its wide   1
sandy bay offers wonderful views of the Isle of Wight in fine weather, together with
the Old Harry Rocks, which stand in the sea at the North End of the beach.

As well as safe swimming, the bay also supports a variety of watersports, including
windsurfing and sailing. Holidaymakers can hire pedalos and motor boats to get   5
out on the water, or take part in organised fishing expeditions. Regular boat trips
also give visitors the chance to see the area's Jurassic coastline, which has been
named England's first World Heritage Site because of its geology.

Boats also visit nearby Poole, Bournemouth and Brownsea Island, which is home
to rare red squirrels. The beach also boasts one of Britain's oldest surviving Punch   10
and Judy shows.

The town itself has plenty to interest tourists. A restored steam railway takes visitors inland to Corfe, with its famous castle. The castle was destroyed during the English Civil War but remains as one of Britain's most striking ruins and is believed to be the inspiration for Kirrin Castle in Enid Blyton's *Famous Five* story *Five on a Treasure Island.*   15

Visitors to Swanage can take part in a variety of sports including golf, tennis, bowls and swimming. There are also miles of stunning cliff top paths nearby for keen walkers or the less energetic can stroll along the town's restored Victorian pier.

Swanage was a fishing and quarrying town until its popularity as a holiday destination grew during the 19th century. Evidence of this development can still be seen in its   20
narrow streets and buildings constructed from local stone. These streets are home to a wide variety of pubs and restaurants to suit all visitors, from locally caught fish and chips to fine French cuisine. There are also many unusual shops selling fossils and gemstones, gifts, jewellery and art. Accommodation on offer ranges from camping, bed and breakfast, and self-catering holiday apartments, right up to five star luxury   25
hotels.

1. Which island can you see from Swanage in fine weather? Circle your answer.

     Isle of Wight   Emerald Isle   Isle of Black

2. What stands in the sea at the North end of the beach? Circle your answer.

     Old Henry Rocks   Old Harry Rocks   Old Harvey Rocks

3. Why has the Jurassic coastline been named a World Heritage site?

_____

4. What is special about the squirrels on Brownsea Island?

_____

5. What does the word *inspiration* mean in line 15?

_____

6. What might keen walkers enjoy?

_____

7–8. Before Swanage first became popular as a holiday destination, what two industries were people employed in?

    _____   _____

9. If you buy fish and chips, where will the fish have been caught?

_____

10. Write a sentence describing what you would most enjoy about a trip to Swanage.

_____

_____ /10

Circle the words or phrases that have come into
the English language in the past 100 years.

11–16.

planet	microchip	mobile phone	book
website	spoon	MP3 player	oven
lamp	plasma TV	supermarket	wheel

/6

Add the **suffix** *ful*, or *ish* to each word to make an **adjective**.

17. care _____   **18.** child _____

19. hope _____   **20.** sorrow _____

21. baby _____   **22.** fool _____   /6

Circle the correct **homophone** to complete each sentence.

23. I (mite might) be able to take piano lessons next year.

24. We are going to (see sea) a show at the theatre on Friday.

25. Sam (threw through) a ball for the kitten to chase.

26. I ate (to two) slices of pizza.

27. We (herd heard) a strange noise outside.

28. I need to (write right) a story about a castle.   /6

Complete these **collective nouns**.

29. a _____ of sheep   **30.** a _____ of cows

31. a _____ of wolves   **32.** a _____ of grapes

33. a _____ of geese   **34.** a _____ of angels   /6

Paper
8

Level 3

Draw lines to match up each bold **verb** with a more powerful alternative.

35.	**walk**	leap
36.	**talk**	beam
37.	**run**	devour
38.	**smile**	saunter
39.	**jump**	sprint
40.	**eat**	chatter

/6

/40

PAPER 8

Dear Diary,

I'm writing this in my new bedroom. It smells of fresh paint and new carpet. This room is exactly how I wanted it. So why doesn't it feel like my room? It sounds really ungrateful, but I want my old room back. It was too small and the pink bunny wallpaper was embarrassing, but it felt like it was mine. This house feels too new, as if it is waiting for another family.

I've been thinking about Hannah and Sally, wondering what they're doing. They'll be at hockey practice tomorrow with the others. They'll probably have a match on Thursday. I don't even know if my new school has a hockey team. Still, I'll find out when I start tomorrow, I suppose.

My new uniform is hanging up on the back of the door. It's scratchy and uncomfortable. I hate the stripy tie and that green skirt is awful! Mum says that I have to give life here a chance; that it's bound to take time to settle in. I know it's hard for her too. She'll be stuck at home with Philip until she finds out about toddler groups for him. She had loads of friends before. Now she'll have to start again. Like me.

Hopefully tomorrow I'll be able to tell you about all my new friends. Maybe I'll get on the hockey team and perhaps my school skirt will look better on me than it does on the hanger!

Love Lucy x

1. What was on the wallpaper in Lucy's old bedroom? Circle your answer.

   puppies   ponies   bunnies

2. What does her new room smell like? Circle your answer.

   varnish and new curtains   fresh paint and new carpet   nail varnish and wood shavings

3–4. Write down two words used to describe how her new uniform feels.

   _____   _____

5. What advice does Lucy's mother give her?

   _____

6. Who is Phillip?

   _____

7. Why is Lucy thinking about her friends?

   _____

   _____

8–10. Write down three hopes that Lucy has for the next day.

   _____

   _____

   _____   /10

Write down the **past tense** for each **present tense verb**.

11. speak _____   **12.** is   _____

13. go   _____   **14.** come   _____

15. find   _____   **16.** catch   _____   /6

Choose a **full stop**, **question mark** or **exclamation mark** to complete each sentence.

17. Do you know where Martin is ___

18. What a beautiful sunset___

19. Mr Monroe is so unfair___

20. The bus was late this morning___

21. Is that a new dress___

22. The boys grabbed their football and ran off___

/6

Add the correct **consonants** to complete the names of different types of fruit.

23. _a _ a _ a

24. a _ _ _ e

25. o _ a _ _ e

26. _ i _ e a _ _ _ e

27. _ e a _

28. _ _ a _ e _

/6

Write down two more words that share the bold letter string with each of these words.

29–30. ni**ght** _____   _____

31–32. t**ear** _____   _____

33–34. sh**ould** _____   _____

/6

Draw lines to separate the **syllables** in each word.

35. c o m p u t e r   **36.**   m a c h i n e r y

37. c u s h i o n   **38.**   h i p p o p o t a m u s

39. b a d g e r   **40.**   m i c r o s c o p e

/6

/40

PAPER 9

On with the show

Falling silently from leaden skies   1
With dancing, drifting clusters
of spiny webs,
winter takes a bow.

Beneath the crystal covering,   5
spring waits in the wings.
Chorus lines of snowdrops waiting
and it's on with the show.

Circle your answers.

1. What do you think is falling in the first verse of the poem?

leaves   rain   snow

2. What colour is a *leaden sky* (line 1)?

grey   blue   black

3. What are the *spiny webs* in line 3?

raindrops   snowflakes   cobwebs

4–6. The poem says that winter takes a bow. Find three other places where the poem makes references to the theatre.

_____

_____

_____

7. What is the *crystal covering* in line 5?

_____

8. What are the *snowdrops* in line 7?

_____ /8

Circle the correct contracted form of the bold words.

9.	**are not**	are'nt	aren't
10.	**he is**	he's	hes'
11.	**they will**	they'll	theyl'l
12.	**should not**	shouldnt'	shouldn't
13.	**you are**	yo'are	you're
14.	**is not**	isn't	isnt'

/6

These words are homonyms. Write a sentence for each word, using a different meaning than before.

15. well _____

16. well _____

17. stamp _____

18. stamp _____

19. coach _____

20. coach _____ /6

Write down the feminine form of these words.

21. king _____

22. brother _____

23. father _____

24. duke _____

25. prince _____

26. uncle _____

/6

TALENT SHOW AUDITION

SINGER?
DANCER?
COMEDIAN?
CONJURER?

If you can do it, we want to see it!

Come to the school hall
at 12.30 on Friday

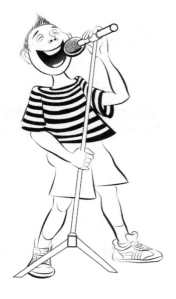

27. What is the poster advertising?

_____

28. What time is it taking place?

_____

29. What does the word *audition* mean?

_____

_____

30. Write down another word with a similar meaning to *conjurer*.

_____   /4

Write down the **plurals** of these **singular nouns**.

31. box _____   **32.** baby _____

33. leaf _____   **34.** beach _____

35. wish _____   **36.** hiss _____   /6

Write an interesting sentence about these topics.

37. Your favourite day of the week

_____

38. An activity you would like to try

_____

39. Your best memory

_____

40. Your first day at your school

_____   /4

/40

PAPER 10

Britain is a nation of chocolate-lovers, munching its way through around 10kg per person each year. After Switzerland, Britain eats more chocolate than anyone else. Most people are so used to chocolate that they are surprised to discover that before the mid-1800s, solid eating chocolate did not exist at all.

The history of chocolate begins in South America, where the Maya and Aztec civilisations developed a spicy drink made from roasted cocoa beans called chocolatl. The drink was made from the beans of the cocoa tree which grew wild in the Amazon basin. Cocoa beans were considered so valuable that as well as being used to make the drink, the beans were used as currency by the Maya. Four beans would buy a pumpkin and ten a rabbit.

After Europeans discovered Mexico during the 1500s, chocolate drinks quickly became popular across Europe. From the mid-1600s chocolate houses began opening in London, offering a range of chocolate drinks along with ale, beer and snacks.

The first solid chocolate bars, for eating, appeared in the mid-1800s. They would probably not be considered tasty by today's standards. At the same time, advances in drinking chocolate production pressed out cocoa butter, which then became available for use in solid chocolate. This made the chocolate tastier.

At first, only plain dark chocolate could be made, but a chocolate-maker from Switzerland experimented with adding first powdered and then condensed milk, resulting in a chocolate bar similar to what people might recognise today.

The range of chocolates available to buy seems to grow each year and the UK now spends more than £3 billion a year on chocolate. Scientists are divided on exactly why we love it so much, but chocolate seems to be here to stay.

1

5

10

15

20

1. Which nation eats the most chocolate? Circle your answer.

    Britain   France   Switzerland

2. What was the earliest chocolate drink called? Circle your answer.

    chocolatl   hotchoc   chocolade

3. What does the word *currency* (line 9) mean?

_____

_____

4–5. Write down two things, apart from chocolate drinks, that might have been served in a chocolate house.

_____   _____

6. When did the first solid eating chocolate appear?

_____

7. What kind of butter made solid chocolate tastier?

_____

8. A chocolate-maker experimented with adding milk to the chocolate. Which country did he come from?

_____

9. How much do British people spend on chocolate each year?

_____

10. Write a sentence explaining why you do, or don't, like chocolate.

_____

_____   **/10**

Use these words to make six **compound words**. Use each word only once.

| cup | pot | match | board | brush | lash |
| eye | stick | hair | foot | ball | tea |

11. _____   **12.** _____

13. _____   **14.** _____

15. _____   **16.** _____   **/6**

Write down a **synonym** for these words.

17. angry _____   **18.** small _____

19. fast _____   **20.** sad _____

21. wet _____   **22.** neat _____   **/6**

Turn these words into **verbs** by adding the **suffix** *en* or *ise.*

23. real_____   **24.** critic_____   **25.** deep_____

26. special_____   **27.** weak_____   **28.** deaf_____

/6

Add *its* or *it's* to complete each sentence.

29. The boat broke clear of _____ moorings.

30. Mum is trying to mend the vase because _____ broken.

31. Our beech tree drops _____ leaves in the autumn.

32. Dad will call us when _____ time for tea.

33. I like maths but _____ hard sometimes.

34. A snake sheds _____ skin as it grows.

/6

Label these sentences **a-f** to arrange them in the right order.

35. _____ We looked everywhere for her.

36. _____ Our dog went missing.

37. _____ Next, the people who found her saw our posters.

38. _____ When we could not find her, we put up posters in our town.

39. _____ Meanwhile, someone had found our dog.

40. _____ Finally, the people brought our dog back to us.

/6

/40

PAPER 11

Wood Lane Primary School Debating Society
Should people be allowed to wear real fur?

"I believe that it is wrong to kill animals just so that we can wear their fur. Animals that are farmed or caught for their fur suffer terribly and there is no need for it to happen. Modern artificial fur looks and feels just like the real thing and it can be made without causing animals to suffer.

Fur is used mainly for fashion, rather than to keep warm, and in any case there are lots of other warm materials we can use to make clothes, like wool and man-made fleece fabrics.

If people stopped buying clothes made with real fur, then the fur trade would disappear completely.

That is why I think people should not wear real fur. Please vote for me, Sam, in the debate."

———————————

"My name is Nina. I believe that there is nothing wrong with wearing animal fur. People have kept warm using fur for thousands of years. Real fur is very warm and beautiful to look at. If people can afford to buy it, why shouldn't they be able to?

Most of us eat meat and I don't see the difference between farming animals for food and farming them for fur.

Also, lots of people have jobs in the fur trade and in the fashion industry. If nobody wore fur these people would have no jobs.

That is why I think people should be able to wear real fur if they want to. Please vote for me in this debate."

1–2. Write down two reasons why Sam thinks that artificial fur is a good idea.

_____

_____

3–4. List two things he suggests we could use instead of fur, to make warm clothes.

_____

_____

5. What does he argue would happen to the fur trade if people stopped buying real fur?

_____

6–7. Write down two advantages of real fur that Nina mentions.

_____

_____

8. In your own words, explain Nina's point about farming for meat and farming for fur.

_____

_____

9–10. Who would you vote for in this debate? Give at least two reasons for your answer.

_____

_____ /10

Write an **antonym** for each word.

11. early _____

12. buy _____

13. float _____

14. hard _____

15. narrow _____

16. first _____

/6

Draw lines to link each word with its **definition**.

17. done with speed   careless

18. full of happiness   really

19. done without attention   graceful

20. genuinely   penniless

21. without money   rapidly

22. moving beautifully   joyful

/6

Write each word in the chart, according to its **prefix**.

23–28. cooperate   misbehave   mistrust   export

coordinate   exchange

mis	co	ex

/6

Add the missing **commas** to each sentence.

29–30. Jack plays cricket football rugby and tennis.

31–32. I have been to Greece Spain France and Italy on holiday.

33. On Saturday Jessica had to clean her room walk the dog and play with her hamster.

34–35. We ordered dough balls pizza garlic bread and salad for lunch.

/7

Write these words again in **alphabetical order**.

house   hoard   hound   hour   hoist

36. _____   **37.** _____

38. _____   **39.** _____

40. _____

/5

/40

PAPER 12

Witness report

It must have been about 12.15pm. I was standing by the lion enclosure with my family. There were lots of people there because the keepers were about to feed the lions.

Some people made room for me so that I could get closer to the wire to see the lions being fed. I could see the keepers opening the gate in the outer fence. They both went inside and closed the gate. I couldn't see whether they locked it again.

The keepers took a large padlock off a small hatch in the inner fence. It wouldn't have been big enough for an adult lion to fit through because even the piece of meat got stuck. The keepers pushed and shoved it and then one of the lions came and started pulling at the meat from inside the enclosure. That must have loosened it because the meat suddenly shot into the enclosure. Two of the adult lionesses started eating the meat straight away and their cubs hung about hoping to get some meat too.

One keeper had started to leave through the outer fence before the other one had closed the hatch. He was watching the lions feeding so he didn't notice that one of the cubs had sneaked up to the hatch and was squeezing through. He dashed through the gate in the outer fence before the keeper could close it.

A few people started to panic and run away but most stayed to watch. The lion seemed curious about people and was running from person to person to have a closer look. The keepers called out, "Stay calm. Don't run or you will scare him."

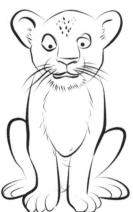

Suddenly a different keeper dashed up with a large, strong net. I couldn't see what happened next because there were people in the way. I could hear the cub snarling and growling and then I saw it back in the cage with the other lions.

Answer these questions.

1. What time of day does the event happen? Circle your answer.

12.15am   12.45am   12.15pm

2. Why does the witness get such a good view of what happened?

_____

_____

Answer booklet English 8–9

Paper 1
1. maths
2. cheese spread
3. Max
4. with coloured chalk on black paper
5. it was rainy
6–7. Joe is writing a story about the autumn.
8. He is making a firework picture and bonfire night takes place in autumn.
9. I would feel surprised and a bit scared.
10. It means to breathe in sharply in surprise or fear.
11. Because he never expected to see a pair of eyes down a drain.
11. green
12. happy
13. huge
14. dark
15. frosty
16. soft
17. candle
18. table
19. cradle
20. bottle
21. stable
22. ankle
23. unhappy
24. disqualify
25. disappear
26. unfair
27. unpack
28. disagree
29–30. door   bell
31–32. cheese   cake
33–34. ear   ring
35. blue
36. green
37. orange
38. pink
39. purple
40. red

Paper 2
1. Europe
2. Because oases have water.
3–5. Any three of the following: Egypt, Libya, Morocco, Chad, Tunisia
6. Because fossils have been found.
7. a hill of sand
8–9. large, flat feet for walking on sand; long eyelashes to keep sound out of their eyes.
10. Because it gets very cold in the desert at night.
11. saw
12. right
13. tap
14. ball
15. train
16. light
17. eggs
18. dishes
19. gloves
20. witches
21. buses
22. zoos
23. The girl climbed the stairs.
24. Flowers grow in the park.
25. A flock of birds flew over our garden.
26. My brother plays basketball for his school.
27. The cat balanced on the fence.
28. Sarah wandered slowly to school.

29–34. pillow, rabbit, fortune, follow, candle, bubble
35. kindly
36. hopeful
37. forgetful
38. actually
39. likely
40. painful

Paper 3
1. to extend the school
2. The buildings were not big enough.
3–4. Because Emily will have to walk for a long time to reach school. Because she will have to cross three major roads.
5. Because they were crumbling.
6–7. Roads will become busier with parents driving to the school. Traffic-calming measures will slow down local traffic.
8. speed bumps
9. Harris Homes
10. In a win-win situation, everybody is better off, so both the schoolchildren and the tax-payers will benefit.
11. there
12. There
13. their
14. there
15. their
16. their
17. low
18. small
19. found
20. full
21. dirty
22. short
23. Ben walked to school.
24. The girls collected shells on the beach.
25. I wished by the wishing well.
26. Mum baked cherry cakes.
27. I switched on the lights at night time.
28. Sally brushed her long hair.
29. table
30. bubble
31. carry
32. happy
33. pepper
34. summer
35. I am
36. she will
37. could not
38. they are
39. he is
40. we will

Paper 4
1. plain
2. flour
3. decoration
4. a flavouring that is not man-made
5. The small amount of salt that can be picked up between the thumb and forefinger.
6. Because it has a golden colour.
7. So the biscuits will not stick.
8. the different foods you mix to make gingerbread men
9. the bowls, spoons, tins etc you need to make gingerbread men
10. biscuit tin
11. France

12. October
13. Monday
14. Sally
15. Europe
16. Liam
17. am
18. is
19. am
20. are
21. are
22. is
23. We were late because the alarm clock was broken.
24. Dad was delighted because he won the football match.
25. Mum made us pizza for tea.
26. I would love to go rock climbing.
27. You must cross the road carefully.
28. Mum and Dad are grumpy when they wake up in the morning.
29. ancient
30. sea
31. concerned
32. street
33. reply
34. home
35. export
36. hopeful
37. heroic
38. winner
39. golden
40. realistic

Paper 5
1. fairytales
2–3. crooked, rickety
4. rotting
5. Because the house is spooky and unusual and they want to know who is living there.
6–7. creaky, squeaky
8. There are bugs in her hair.
9. She was about to have dinner.
10. She wants to put the children in her soup.
11–16. camel, come, giant, grape, sausage, soil
17–22. First, Grandad filled little pots with compost, before using a pencil to make a little hole in the soil. Next, he dropped a seed into each hole, then gently covered the seed with compost. After that, he watered each pot carefully and finally placed them on the windowsill in the sunlight.
23. childhood
24. knighthood
25. friendship
26. boyhood
27. ownership
28. neighbourhood
29. partnership
30. membership
31. "What a beautiful picture!" said the teacher.
32. Dad called up the stairs, "Have you seen my keys?"
33. Poppy shouted, "Great goal!"
34. "We'll be late if we don't hurry!" warned Mum.
35. the dog's paw
36. the woman's car
37. a cat's tail
38. the girl's foot
39. a town's roads
40. the boy's nose

1

Paper 6

1. monkey
2. kuyu
3. Because he is sick of eating salty fish.
4–5. crafty, puzzled
6. king
7. He is afraid because he knows that the shark wants his heart.
8. He tells the shark that he left his heart in a tree at home so he needs to go back and get it.
9. 9 days
10. I think the monkey is wiser because he manages to trick the shark into taking him home safely.
11. Anna wrote as neatly as she could, not smudging the ink at all.
12. Tail wagging wildly, the puppy chased the ball.
13. Not finding any boots she liked, Nina bought some shoes instead.
14. When nobody answered the phone, Max left a message.
15. kindly
16. prettily
17. actually
18. daintily
19. fully
20. dizzily
21. rudely
22. gracefully
23. Mark
24. 3
25. Paulo
26. Because he is the oldest.
27. piglet
28. duckling
29. gosling
30. kitten
31. signet
32. foal
33. cub
34. joey
35. while
36. when
37. because
38. so
39. but
40. before

Paper 7

1. Isle of Wight
2. Old Harry Rocks
3. because of its geology
4. they are rare red squirrels
5. a thing that gives someone the idea for something
6. miles of cliff-top walks
7–8. fishing, quarrying
9. in the sea off Swanage
10. Answers will vary.
11–16. microchip, mobile phone, MP3 player, website, plasma TV, supermarket
17. careful
18. childish
19. hopeful
20. sorrowful
21. babyish
22. foolish
23. might
24. see
25. threw
26. two
27. heard
28. write
29. flock

30. herd
31. pack
32. bunch
33. gaggle
34. host
35. saunter
36. chatter
37. sprint
38. beam
39. leap
40. devour

Paper 8

1. bunnies
2. fresh paint and new carpet
3–4. scratchy, uncomfortable
5. She advises her to give life there a chance.
6. Lucy's younger brother
7. Because they have moved house.
8–10. to make new friends; to get on the hockey team; that her skirt will look better on her than on the hanger
11. spoke
12. was
13. went
14. came
15. found
16. caught
17. ?
18. !
19. !
20. .
21. ?
22. .
23. banana
24. apple
25. orange
26. pineapple
27. pear
28. grapes
29–34. Possible answers include:
29–30. tight, fright
31–32. fear, year
33–34. could, would
35. com/pu/ter
36. mach/in/er/y
37. cush/ion
38. hipp/o/pot/am/us
39. badg/er
40. mi/cro/scope

Paper 9

1. snow
2. grey
3. snowflakes
4–6. spring waits in the wings, chorus lines, on with the show
7. snow
8. flowers
9. aren't
10. he's
11. they'll
12. shouldn't
13. you're
14. isn't
15–20. Answers will vary.
21. queen
22. sister
23. mother
24. duchess
25. princess
26. aunt
27. a talent show
28. 12.30pm
29. An event where people show what they can do to see if they are good enough to enter the talent show.

30. magician
31. boxes
32. babies
33. leaves
34. beaches
35. wishes
36. hisses
37–40. Answers will vary.

Paper 10

1. Switzerland
2. chocolatl
3. money
4–5. Any two from: ale, beer, snacks
6. mid-1800s
7. cocoa butter
8. Switzerland
9. £3 billion
10. Answers will vary.
11. cupboard
12. eyelash
13. matchstick
14. football
15. teapot
16. hairbrush
17–22. Possible answers include:
17. cross
18. tiny
19. quick
20. unhappy
21. damp
22. tidy
23. realise
24. criticise
25. deepen
26. specialise
27. weaken
28. deafen
29. its
30. it's
31. its
32. it's
33. it's
34. its
35–40. b, a, e, c, d, f

Paper 11

1–2. it looks like the real thing, it can be made without harming animals
3–4. wool, man-made fleece fabric
5. it would disappear
6–7. it is very warm, it looks beautiful
8. she argues that there is no difference between farming animals for meat and farming them for fur
9–10. Answers will vary.
11–16. Possible answers include:
11. late
12. sell
13. sink
14. soft/easy
15. wide
16. last
17. rapidly
18. joyful
19. careless
20. really
21. penniless
22. graceful
23–28.

mis	co	ex
misbehave	cooperate	export
mistrust	coordinate	exchange

29–30. Jack plays cricket, football, rugby and tennis.
31–32. I have been to Greece, Spain, France and Italy on holiday.

33. On Saturday Jessica had to walk the dog, clean out the rabbits and play with her hamster.
34–35. We ordered dough balls, pizza, garlic bread and salad for lunch.
36–40. hoard, hoist, hound, hour, house

Paper 12
1. 12.15pm
2. Adults made room for them so they could see the lions being fed.
3. the meat got stuck in the hatch
4–5. They leave the hatch open, one keeper opens the outer gate before the hatch is closed.
6. An adult lion could not have escaped because the hatch was too small.
7. The cub was not dangerous because most people are not afraid of it and the keepers were worried that the people would scare the cub, not that the cub would harm the people.
8–9. whether the keeper locked the gate; how the cub got back into the cage
10. The lion cub was caught by the keeper in the net and put back in the cage.
11. five boys' test papers
12. the girl's bag
13. six birds' wings
14. three dogs' tails
15. the five teachers' desks
16. three cars' engines
17. although
18. so
19. but
20. and
21. if
22. because
23–28.

common nouns	proper nouns
mouse	Paris
week	Christmas
class	Jennifer

29. A large, black cat was curled up on the chair.
30. The cake was smothered with sweet, sticky, pink icing.
31. Laura's hair, tangled and windswept, stood out in all directions.
32. We left footprints in the cold, crisp, white snow.
33. Luke rode by on his blue, shiny new bike.
34. The garden was full of bright, colourful flowers.
35. though
36. twice
37. shout
38. sausage
39. earn
40. height

Paper 13
1. school
2. They didn't like the school food.
3. sports socks and sweaty trainers
4. Jack
5. Because they can do it later or Mum might do them with the dinner things.
6. Because she is tired from work.
7. Because it is her birthday cake.

8. Ben
9–10. Answers will vary.
11. better
12. darker
13. neater
14. quicker
15. sweeter
16. warmer
17–20. Possible answers include: ceiling, receive, circle, circus
21–22. Answers will vary.
23. hoping
24. dinner
25. bitter
26. lady
27. tapping
28. supper
29. "Hurry up!" called Mum.
30. "Where are my hockey boots?" asked Saffron.
31. "Does everyone have enough to eat?" asked Dad.
32. "That tickles!" giggled Sophie.
33. "Get out of my room!" shouted Mark, angrily.
34. "Which way is the swimming pool?" asked Lucy.
35. environment
36. statement
37. fitness
38. government
39. kindness
40. illness

Paper 14
1. 20 minutes
2. the footpath is narrow
3. 10 minutes
4. The shop sells great sweets.
5–6. footbridge, zebra crossing
7. blue
8. reserved for people walking
9. 3.00pm
10. to play football
11–16. sheep, fish, aircraft, buffalo, salmon, traffic
17–22. Answers will vary.
23. weakling
24. droplet
25. bracelet
26. sapling
27. leaflet
28. dumpling
29–30. I scored four goals for our team.
31–32. Sam knew straight away that he would like the new boy.
33–34. Chloe ran inside because she did not want to be stung by the bee.
35–36. I would love to stay up late but I know that Mum will say no.
37–40. Poppy likes dogs.
Sally doesn't like drawing pictures.
Poppy does not like playing netball.
Sally enjoys PE lessons.

Paper 15
1. A song that sends people to sleep.
2–3. Barney is a dog. He has fur, and he does not like cats.
4. Because it is raining.
5. to the farm
6. Because none of the boxes smelled of food.
7. sausages
8. the sound of sausages cooking
9. breakfast time
10. He is about to steal the sausages.
11. promotion

12. translation
13. reaction
14. creation
15. education
16. conclusion
17. My friend kept chickens.
18. I could ice skate really well.
19. I saw my grandparents every weekend.
20. Faith wrote secrets in her diary.
21. I bought a magazine each Friday.
22. I ran faster than anyone else in my class.
23. we're
24. I'll
25. they're
26. you've
27. it'll
28. would've
29. he
30. them
31. we
32. they
33. us
34. me
35–37. Answers will vary.
38–40. Answers will vary.

Paper 16
1. distant or isolated
2. By charging each other less than they should.
3. A violent storm blew up.
4. The door had blown in and half of the roof had gone.
5. Because he had just made a lot of money selling his work, so he didn't need to work any more.
6. Because he had been helping people who couldn't afford to pay him.
7. Their houses are cold and damp.
8. The carpenter could have prevented some people from becoming ill by fixing their houses so that they were not cold and damp.
9. The fact that the carpenter can pay will not make a difference to how quickly his son is treated because the doctor does not mind whether or not his patients can pay him.
10. The carpenter became greedy when he became rich, so he wouldn't help his neighbours any more.
11. sword
12. woman
13. wolf
14. wool
15. worm
16. two
17–20. Possible answers include:
17. I clambered over the slippery rocks at the foot of the cliff.
18. Paul dozed restlessly in the chair by the fire.
19. Maria gazed out of the window at the view.
20. Peter smashed the piggy bank to see what was inside.
21–28.

phone	oct	vent	press
telephone	octopus	invent	pressure
megaphone	octagon	prevent	impress

29. pitiful
30. running

3

31. daring
32. stylish
33. beautiful
34. childish
35. bull
36. drake
37. grandfather
38. nephew
39. lady
40. husband

Paper 17

1. a shopping centre
2. 10
3. 9.00am
4–5. Any two of: jugglers, acrobats, stilt walkers
6. No, some are worried about the roads around the centre.
7. Disruption means something that interferes with or spoils the normal routine.
8. To make up for the inconvenience the people of the town have had to put up with.
9. a digger which damaged gas pipes and a water main
10. Because they are worried that the new car park will not be big enough for the extra traffic.
11–15. Possible answers include:
11. kitchen
12. It
13. sauntered
14. dewy
15. lightly
16. its
17. It's
18. it's
19. its
20. its

ible	able
edible	reliable
horrible	adorable
possible	enjoyable
responsible	valuable

21–28.
29–30. Our cat, who hates water, got soaked in the rain.
31. Running for the bus, I tripped and fell.
32–33. On the school trip we tried canoeing, abseiling, climbing and raft-building.
34. After a good wash, the car looked like new.
35. I needed to buy flour, sugar and eggs to make the cake.
36. left
37. fair
38. wave
39. jam
40. book

Paper 18

1. sofa
2. 2
3. It was the wrong colour.
4. Because young children can make a mess.
5. Because it does not match the rest of his furniture.
6. He rang the store to complain.
7. No, because they only wanted to buy one beige sofa and the mistake is not their fault.

8–9. disappointed, angry
10. He wants a full refund.
11–18.

add er	add est
taller	tallest
bigger	biggest
hotter	hottest
shorter	shortest

19–22. Answers will vary.
23. transatlantic
24. telephone
25. television
26. transparent
27. translate
28. telescope
29–34. Possible answers include:
29. cough
30. near
31. soup
32. launch
33. spice
34. wait
35–40. Possible answers include:
35. We relaxed in the warm sun.
36. Pippa is terrified of the dark.
37. The old house was spooky.
38. We chose a huge Christmas tree.
39. Dad was furious because I was late home.
40. It was chilly last night.

Paper 19

1. she does
2. 3
3. No, because he had only seen cows in pictures and has come from London.
4. jostled
5. He could be crushed between two cows or trampled beneath their hooves
6. She means that they will be gentle because lambs are gentle.
7–8. grass-scented sighs; air smelt fresh and clear
9. Because they were not safe in the air-raids in London.
10. during World War II
11. autograph
12. automobile
13. bicycle
14. bifocal
15. autobiography
16. bilingual
17. bimonthly
18. autopilot
19–22. Landing in Egypt, we couldn't believe how hot it was.
23–28. Possible answers include:
23. valuable
24. in the end
25. the letters of the alphabet except a,e,i,o and u
26. having courage
27. nearby
28. a room or building containing many books
29–34. Sentences will vary.
35–40. Possible answers include:
35. handbag
36. railway
37. airport
38. motorbike
39. windmill
40. playground

Paper 20

1. a holiday which combines a cruise with a stay in a hotel
2. A trip to visit a place or attraction.
3–4. Any two of: Valley of the Kings, Luxor Temple, Karnak Temple, Aswan High Dam
5. So that they can speak Egyptian to local Egyptians and also answer the questions of English-speaking guests.
6. Because Egypt is a hot country.
7–8. Any two of: Luxor Museum, sound and light show, Colossi of Memnon
9. To save them from being flooded during the construction of the Aswan Dam.
10. No, unlimited use of the spa is included in the price.
11. stationary
12. personal
13. atomic
14. realistic
15. dictionary
16. seasonal
17–32. Possible answers include:
17–18. curious, serious
19–20. social, artificial
21–22. rough, though
23–28. Possible answers include:
23. The storm was approaching rapidly so we walked more quickly towards home.
24. The funny clown told us a hilarious joke.
25. John is unkind to the younger children and mean to his sister.
26. I cut up an onion while Dad chopped a pepper to go in the chilli.
27. Jenny was happy with her present and Max was delighted with his.
28. The pretty princess had beautiful hair.
29–34. Possible answers include:

29.	a sunset	fiery golden ball
30.	a lion	ferocious predator
31.	a traffic jam	winding into the distance like a snake
32.	a waterfall	a wall of shimmering water
33.	a beach	a sandy strip, yellow against the blue sea
34.	a roller coaster	a winding framework curling like metallic ribbon

35–40. Possible answers include:
35. "Your picture is great!" said Mark, admiringly.
36. The stars twinkled brightly in the inky sky.
37. The boys gobbled up the chips hungrily.
38. I wrote the answers neatly on the test paper.
39. "Hello!" called the twins, cheerfully.
40. James built the model ship carefully.

3. What happened to the meat when the keepers tried to feed the lions?

_____

_____

4–5. List two mistakes that the keepers made that allowed the cub to escape.

_____

_____

6. Would it have been possible for an adult lion to escape in the same way? Give a reason for your answer.

_____

_____

7. Do you think the cub was dangerous? Use evidence from the text to support your answer.

_____

_____

8–9. List two things in the statement that the witness doesn't see clearly.

_____

_____

10. How do you think the lion cub got back into the cage?

_____

_____

/10

Add the **apostrophe** in the correct place.

11. five boys test papers

12. the girls bag

13. six birds wings

14. three dogs tails

15. the five teachers desks

16. three cars engines

/6

Choose a suitable **conjunction** from the box to complete each sentence.

and   although   because   if   so   but

17. Katie shared her lunch _____ she was hungry.

18. I worked hard _____ I would do well in my test.

19. I loved the shoes _____ the shop did not have them in my size.

20. I passed the ball to Nick _____ he scored a goal.

21. I can watch my favourite TV programme _____ I finish my homework in time.

22. Mum was angry _____ my room was in a mess.

/6

Complete this table by sorting these words into **common nouns** and **proper nouns**.

Paris   mouse   Christmas   week   Jennifer   class

23–28.

common nouns	proper nouns

/6

Underline the **adjectival phrase** in each sentence.

29. A large, black cat was curled up on the chair.

30. The cake was smothered with sweet, sticky, pink icing.

31. Laura's hair, tangled and wind-swept, stood out in all directions.

32. We left footprints in the cold, crisp, white snow.

33. Luke rode by on his blue, shiny, new bike.

34. The garden was full of bright, colourful flowers.

/6

Draw lines to match up the pairs of words that have the same letter string but a different sound.

35.	c**ough**	shout
36.	not**ice**	sausage
37.	fo**ur**	though
38.	**au**nt	height
39.	h**ear**	twice
40.	w**eight**	earn

/6

/40

PAPER 13

Scene 2

Jack and Ben come in from school. They are in the kitchen. Jack opens the fridge door.

Ben: I'm starving!

Jack: Me too! That pasta bake at lunchtime was disgusting.
          What do they put in school food?

Ben: I reckon they boil up all the sports socks and sweaty trainers in lost property! Hey
          do you want some of this cake?

Ben takes out a chocolate cake on a plate.

Jack: Do you think we should?

Ben: Oh come on! It's only a cake. I'm having some, even if you don't.

Jack: Oh go on then, just a small bit.

The boys quickly eat all of the cake.

Jack: We'd better wash up these plates.

Ben: No, don't worry about it. We'll do it later. If we're lucky, Mum'll do them with the dinner plates. No sense making work for ourselves.

The boys leave as Mum comes in from work. She is carrying heavy shopping and looks tired.

Mum: Hello boys. Good day?

Ben calls from offstage: It was OK mum.

Mum: (*angrily*) Ben, Jack, come here!

Mum is holding up the cake plate as the boys come into the kitchen

Mum: What's this?

Ben: We were hungry.

Jack: We were going to wash up the plates, honest!

Mum: That was my birthday cake! You've eaten the whole thing!

1. Where have the boys come in from? Circle your answer.

   a football match   the shops   school

2. Why are they hungry? Circle your answer.

   they forgot their   they didn't like   they didn't eat
     packed lunch   the school food   any breakfast

3. What does Ben think they put in the school food?

   _____

4. Who isn't sure whether they should eat the cake?

   _____

5. Why does Ben say they shouldn't wash up the plates?

   _____

   _____

6. Why might Mum not be in a very good mood, even before she sees the cake plates?

   _____

   _____

7. Why do you think Mum is angry about the cake?

_____

_____

8. Which of the two boys do you think has behaved the worst?

_____

_____

9–10. Write down two things you might happen in the next scene?

_____

_____

_____ /10

Find and underline an **adjective** in each sentence that ends with *er*.

11. I want my project to be better than my last one.

12. Now that is it autumn, the evenings are much darker.

13. My homework is neater than I have managed before.

14. Dan ran the race quicker than the rest of the team.

15. Adding sugar to teak makes it taste sweeter.

16. I changed my thin jacket for a warmer coat. /6

Write down four words which contain a soft *c*, e.g. cinema

17. _____ **18.** _____

19. _____ **20.** _____ /4

Choose two of your words and write a sentence containing each one.

21. _____

22. _____ /2

Underline the correct word in each set of brackets to complete the sentences.

23. I am (hoping hopping) to get a guitar for my birthday.

24. Mum and Dad love holding (diner dinner) parties.

25. We don't eat orange peel because it is (biter bitter).

26. I stood up on the bus to let an old (lady laddy) sit down.

27. The tree branch was (taping tapping) against my bedroom window.

28. We had cheese on toast for (supper super).

/6

Add the **speech marks** to these sentences.

29. Hurry up! called Mum.

30. Where are my hockey boots? asked Saffron.

31. Does everyone have enough to eat? asked Dad.

32. That tickles! giggled Sophie.

33. Get out of my room! shouted Mark, angrily.

34. Which way is the swimming pool? asked Lucy.

/6

Add the **suffix** *ness* or *ment* to each word.

35. environ_____

36. state_____

37. fit_____

38. govern_____

39. kind_____

40. ill_____

/6

/40

PAPER 14

Dear Harry

I am very glad you can come and play for the team at the weekend. If your parents can't drop you off, it only takes 20 minutes to walk from your house. Here are the directions.

Turn right out of your gate. Walk to the end of your road, then turn right again into Boundary Road. Half way down, cross at the zebra crossing and turn into Mill Lane. The pavement is rather narrow so be careful if there is a lot of traffic.

When you get to the end of Mill Lane there is a public footpath. It is a short-cut through to Albion Road which should save you 10 minutes. At the end of the footpath turn left along Albion Road until you get to a corner with a sweet shop. (Bring some money because this shop sells great sweets!)

After the sweet shop, cross the side-road and carry on along Albion Road until it joins Church Street. This is a very busy road so carry on until you get to the footbridge and cross there. Look for a blue house. There's a path between it and the neighbouring house that will bring you out by the shopping centre. This whole area is pedestrianised so you don't need to worry about traffic!

I'm sure you know how to get to the park from there. It's about five minutes walk down the High Street, then left by the baker shop.

I'll be there from about 3pm and kick-off is at 3.30pm. Don't forget your footie boots!

See you on Saturday,

Jacob

Circle your answers.

1. How long should it take Harry to walk to the park?

　　10 minutes　　　　25 minutes　　　　20 minutes

2. Why should Harry be careful in Mill Lane?

　　the road is busy　　　the footpath is narrow　　　a fierce dog lives there

3. Jacob suggests a short cut through to Albion Road. How much time should that save Harry?

　　10 minutes　　　　20 minutes　　　　5 minutes

Answer these questions.

4. Why does Jacob suggest that Harry should bring some money?

_____

5–6. List two different ways mentioned in the directions to cross roads safely.

_____

_____

7. What colour is the house Jacob should look for?

_____

8. If a pedestrian is someone walking rather than driving, what do you think the word *pedestrianised* means?

_____

_____

9. What time will Jacob be at the park on Saturday?

_____

10. Why are they meeting at the park?

_____   /10

Circle the words which do not change in the **plural**.

11–16. sheep   mouse   kite   fish   aircraft   cow

buffalo   salmon   kitten   traffic   house   nation   /6

Write a sentence containing each **verb** and **adverb** pair.

17. walked quickly

_____

18. walked slowly

_____

19. sang beautifully

_____

20. sang terribly

_____

21. worked carefully

_____

22. worked carelessly

_____ /6

Add *ling* or *let* to each word to make a **diminutive**.

23. weak_____   **24.** drop_____   **25.** brace_____

26. sap_____   **27.** leaf_____   **28.** dump_____   /6

Put the pairs of **homophones** in the correct place in each sentence.

29–30. I scored _____ goals _____ our team. (for four)

31–32. Sam _____ straight away that he would like the _____ boy. (knew new)

33–34. Chloe ran inside because she did not want to _____ stung by the _____.
(bee be)

35–36. I would love to stay up late but I _____ that Mum will say _____.
(no know)   /8

Read the text, then underline the sentences that are true.

Poppy has a brother. She loves all animals, drawing pictures and writing stories. She doesn't like any sport.

Sally has two sisters. She is good at gymnastics and loves going to parties. She doesn't like art.

37–40. Poppy likes dogs.   Sally has a brother.

Sally doesn't like drawing pictures.   Poppy has two sisters.

Poppy does not like playing netball.   Sally enjoys PE lessons.   /4

/40

PAPER 15

The steady sound of the train worked like a lullaby on Barney. When he woke up,   1
he could see pinpricks of daylight around the edge of the carriage door. He felt
the train slow down, and heard voices outside. The door slid open and faces
peered in.

Barney didn't wait to find out whether they were friendly or not. Growling, he   5
leapt off the train and ran. Hearing the train pull out the station behind him and
pick up speed, Barney decided he was safe for now. He slowed to a trot.

It had started to rain heavily and Barney's fur was wet through. Shaking himself
briskly, Barney looked around for a place to shelter. There were houses up ahead
and one had an old garage at the front. It didn't look very cosy, or very safe for   10
that matter, but the door was open a little and Barney crept inside.

Out of the rain, Barney had time to think. In this weather, finding drinking water
wouldn't be a problem but he'd had nothing to eat since the previous morning.
If he was going to find his way back to his farm he would need to find some food
first. He looked around him. The garage was full of cardboard boxes. Some had   15
old car parts sticking out of the top. Others were sealed shut with thick brown
tape. None of them smelled of food but at least there was no sign of any cats.

Barney ventured out of the garage. A delicious smell wafted past him. Sausages!
Barney followed the smell around the back of the garage and along a winding
path to the back of the house. The kitchen door was open and Barney could   20
hear sizzling from inside. Mouth watering, Barney crept up to the back door and
peered inside. There was the cooker and there was the frying pan. Judging by
the smell coming from the pan, the food was nearly ready. Best of all, there was
nobody guarding his breakfast!

Answer these questions.

1. What does the word *lullaby* (line 1) mean?

_____

2–3 Who or what do you think Barney is? Give two pieces of evidence from the text to explain
how you know.

_____

_____

4. Why wouldn't it be a problem for Barney to find drinking water?

_____

5. Where is Barney trying to get back to?

_____

6. How did Barney know there was no food in the garage?

_____

7. What can Barney smell when he leaves the garage?

_____

8. What is the sizzling sound that Barney can hear?

_____

9. What time of day is it in the story?

_____

10. What is Barney about to do when the story extract ends?

_____ **/10**

Add the **suffix** *ion* to each word. You may need
to alter the spelling of the word slightly first.

11. promote + ion =   _____

12. translate + ion =   _____

13. react + ion =   _____

14. create + ion =   _____

15. educate + ion =   _____

16. conclude + ion =   _____   **/6**

Write these sentences again in the **past tense**.

17. My friend keeps chickens.

_____

18. I can ice skate really well.

_____

19. I see my grandparents every weekend.

_____

20. Faith writes secrets in her diary.

_____

21. I buy a magazine each Friday.

_____

22. I run faster than anyone else in my class.

_____   /6

Write these pairs of words as **contractions**.

23. we are _____   24. I will _____

25. they are _____   26. you have _____

27. it will _____   28. would have _____   /6

Add a suitable **personal pronoun** to complete each sentence.

29. Dad hunted high and low because _____ could not find his car keys.

30. My friends are coming over later so I can help _____ with their homework.

31. My brother and I brushed our teeth because _____ were going to the dentist.

32. My cousins like coming to stay because _____ love exploring the city.

33. It was cold playing in the snow so Mum made _____ some hot chocolate.

34. My auntie bought _____ a new outfit for my birthday.

/6

Write a sentence to match each sentence ending.

35. _____ ?

36. _____ !

37. _____ .

/3

Write an **adjectival phrase** to describe these things.

38. a snowy scene _____

39. fireworks _____

40. a beach _____

/3

/40

PAPER 16

The proud carpenter

Many years ago there lived a poor carpenter. He worked hard and his work was   1
good but the people in his remote village never had enough money to pay him,
so he always charged them less than he should. The villagers all helped each
other in this way. All were good workers who charged less than they could, to
help their neighbours.   5

One day, a rich merchant passed through the village. He admired the carpenter's
beautiful work so much that he offered to buy it all, at a very high price. The
delighted carpenter agreed and sat down to count his money.

That night a violent storm blew up. Many of the village houses were damaged. At first
light the carpenter's neighbour, who was a doctor, knocked at his door.   10

"My door has blown in and half of my roof has gone," he said. "Please help me."

The carpenter remembered the praise of the merchant and the pile of money he
had paid.

"What can you pay me?" asked the carpenter.

"My friend, I have no money," he replied. "When people are sick I try to heal them   15
but nobody has money to pay me. You know how it is."

The carpenter grew angry. "I am a great carpenter. Yesterday I sold all of my work at
a high price. If you can't pay me then I won't help you."

Throughout the day, other neighbours came to ask the carpenter for help. Each time
he sent them away with the same message. Some time later, the carpenter's son became   20
very ill. The carpenter immediately called on his neighbour, the doctor. His wife answered
the door.

"I'm sorry," she said. "Since the storm, the villagers' damaged homes are cold and damp.
Their children are sick. My husband is trying to heal them."

"But I can pay!" argued the carpenter.   25

The doctor's wife shrugged. "When he gets back I'll tell him you called, but he's very
busy. You know how it is."

1. What is the meaning of the word *remote* (line 2)?

_____

2. How did the villagers manage to buy what they needed from each other?

_____

_____

3. A rich merchant bought the carpenter's work. What happened to the village that night?

_____

_____

4. What damage was done to the house of the carpenter's neighbour?

_____

_____

5. Explain in your own words why the carpenter would not help.

_____

_____

6. Why couldn't the doctor pay for the repairs to his house?

_____

_____

7. Some time later, more people in the village become ill. What reason does the doctor's wife give for this?

_____

_____

8. Do you think that the carpenter could have prevented some of the villagers from becoming ill? Give a reason for your answer.

_____

_____

9. Do you think the fact that the carpenter can pay the doctor will make a difference to how quickly his son is treated? Give a reason for your answer.

_____

_____

10. What do you think was the main mistake the carpenter made?

_____

_____ /10

Write a word that contains the *wo* letter string for each picture.

11. _____

12. _____

13. _____

14. _____

15. _____

16. _____

/6

Write these sentences again, replacing the
bold **verb** with a more powerful one.

17. I **climbed** over the slippery rocks at the foot of the cliff.

_____

_____

18. Paul **slept** restlessly in the chair by the fire.

_____

_____

19. Maria **looked** out of the window at the view.

_____

_____

20. Peter **broke** the piggy bank to see what was inside.

_____

_____ /4

Write these words in the chart according to their **word roots**.

21–28.   telephone   octagon   prevent   impress

pressure   megaphone   octopus   invent

phone	oct	vent	press

/8

Add the **suffix** *ish*, *ing* or *ful* to make **adjectives**.
You may need to alter the spellings.

29. pity   +   _____   =   _____

30. run   +   _____   =   _____

31. dare   +   _____   =   _____

32. style   +   _____   =   _____

33. beauty +   _____   =   _____

34. child   +   _____   =   _____

/6

Draw lines to match up the pairs of masculine and feminine words.

35.	cow	nephew
36.	duck	lady
37.	grandmother	bull
38.	neice	husband
39.	lord	drake
40.	wife	grandfather

/6

/40

PAPER 17

Ready, steady, shop!

High Heston is counting down to the grand opening of The Steeples this Friday. 1
    The long-awaited shopping centre is home to the biggest high street names together with restaurants and bars, a bowling alley and 10-screen cinema. The centre will be the largest in the region and is bringing hundreds of new jobs to the town.

    The grand opening kicks off at 9am this Friday when the Town Mayor will officially open the centre. 5
Throughout the day, shoppers will be entertained by bands and teams of jugglers, stilt-walkers and acrobats. The cinema complex is offering cut-price tickets all day Friday and several of the bars and cafes will be running special offers. On Saturday there will be puppet shows and face-painting for the children.

    Centre manager Neil Barton explains: "High Heston has waited five long years for the shopping centre to open. We know that there has been some disruption to road-users during construction so we 10
wanted to put on a big show for the opening, to thank people for their patience."

    The Steeples has not been without its critics. Local residents opposed the development when plans were first submitted, arguing that the roads in and around High Heston would not cope with the additional traffic the centre would bring.

    Earlier in the year the centre of town was brought to a standstill when a digger preparing foundations 15
for the car park damaged gas pipes and a water main. It will take a lot to make local residents forget the three weeks of disruption they endured. Many are worried that the new car park will not be big enough for the shoppers visiting the centre from out of town, leading to more misery on the roads.

    So will it all have been worth it? High Heston residents can decide for themselves, from Friday.

Circle your answers.

1. What is The Steeples?

a church   a shopping centre   a car park

2. How many screens does the cinema have?

10   5   12

3. What time does the centre open on Friday?

9.30am   9.00pm   9.00am

Answer these questions.

4–5. List two things that will entertain shoppers on opening day.

_____

_____

6. Were all the residents of High Heston excited about the shopping centre when it was first announced? Explain your answer.

_____

_____

7. What does the word *disruption* (line 10) mean?

_____

_____

8. What reason does the manager give for wanting to have an exciting launch day?

_____

_____

9. What brought the town centre to a standstill earlier in the year?

_____

_____

10. What are some people still worried about now that the centre is completed?

_____

_____

_____ **/10**

Find and write down one example of each
word type from this piece of writing.

Hearing voices in the kitchen, the tabby cat arched its back and sprang lightly down off the
fence. It sauntered lazily across the dewy grass towards its cat-flap.

11. noun _____

12. pronoun _____

13. verb _____

14. adjective _____

15. adverb _____ **/5**

Add *it's* or *its* to complete each sentence.

16. It's funny when our puppy chases _____ tail.

17. _____ too late to take care of something when it's already broken.

18. I don't like cabbage because _____ slimy.

19. The rabbit scurried back down _____ burrow.

20. The book was muddy and _____ pages were torn. **/5**

Sort these words into the table, according to whether they have the **suffix** *ible* or *able*.

21–28. edible   reliable   horrible   possible

adorable   enjoyable   responsible   valuable

ible	able

/8

Add **commas** to these sentences.

29–30. Our cat who hates water got soaked in the rain.

31. Running for the bus I tripped and fell.

32–33. On the school trip we tried canoeing abseiling climbing and raft-building.

34. After a good wash the car looked like new.

35. I needed to buy flour sugar and eggs to make the cake.

/7

Underline the **homonym** in each sentence that is used twice, each with a different meaning.

36. After we left the cinema we turned left and headed for home.

37. It isn't fair that I can't go on the big rides at the fair.

38. I saw Dad wave frantically just before the huge wave knocked me off my surfboard.

39. We sat for hours in the traffic jam, eating crisps and jam sandwiches.

40. We enjoyed reading the book so much that we couldn't wait to book tickets to see the film.

/5

/40

PAPER 18

Greg Smith,
23 Laurel Lane,
Chester
CH14 4PV

The Manager,
The Sofa Centre,
Main Street,
Chester

12th March

Dear Sir,

I am writing to complain about the sofa I bought from your store, which was delivered yesterday.

To begin with, the sofa should have been delivered last Tuesday. I took the day off work to wait for the delivery man but he did not come. I had to take another day off yesterday and then he didn't come until 6.30pm, so I could have gone to work after all.

When I unwrapped the sofa I realised that it is the wrong colour. I ordered beige but this sofa is white. We have young children so a white sofa is hardly practical. It also does not match our other furniture.

I telephoned the store this morning to complain and was told that I would have to wait three months for a replacement sofa. The manager also said that if we used the white sofa while we are waiting, we will have to pay for both sofas! What are we supposed to sit on for the next three months?

I am very disappointed by the service I have received from your company and angry that we will have to wait for a replacement sofa when the mistake was not our fault.

I would like a full refund of all the money we have paid, so that we can buy the sofa from someone else.

Yours faithfully,

Greg Smith

Circle your answers.

1. What is Mr Smith complaining about?

a sofa   a delivery man   a shop

2. How many days did Mr Smith take off work to wait for the sofa to be delivered?

1   2   3

3. When he unwrapped it, what was wrong with it?

    it was too big   it was damaged   it was the wrong colour

4. Why is a white sofa not practical when you have young children?

_____

5. Why else does he not want a white sofa?

_____

6. How did Mr Smith find out that he would have to wait three months for the right sofa?

_____

7. Do you think it is fair that the Smith family will have to pay for both sofas if they sit on the white one while they are waiting for the replacement? Explain your answer.

_____

_____

8–9. Write down two words from the letter that describe how Mr Smith feels.

_____

10. What does Mr Smith want from the sofa company?

_____

/10

Complete this **adjective** table. You may need to double the final letter of some words before adding the **suffix**.

11–18

tall big hot short

add *er*	ad *est*

/8

Write an interesting sentence about:

19. your school

_____

_____

20. your favourite food

_____

_____

21. a hobby you have

_____

_____

22. a place you have been on holiday

_____

_____ /4

Add the **prefix** *trans* or *tele* to each word.

23. _____ atlantic

24. _____ phone

25. _____ vision

26. _____ parent

27. _____ late

28. _____ scope /6

Write a word that shares the bold letter string.

29. en**ough** _____

30. l**ear**n _____

31. j**ou**rney _____

32. s**au**ce _____

33. r**ice** _____

34. f**air** _____

/6

Write these sentences again, replacing
the bold word with a better **synonym**.

35. We relaxed in the **hot** sun.

_____

36. Pippa is **frightened** of the dark.

_____

37. The old house was **creepy**.

_____

38. We chose a **big** Christmas tree.

_____

39. Dad was **angry** because I was late home.

_____

40. It was **cold** last night.

_____

/6

/40

Chapter 2

Very early the next morning, Mrs Bowers took us out and showed us the cowsheds, where lines of cows waited with bulging udders for milking to begin. She explained that with Mr Bowers and their two sons away fighting, she had to manage the milking herself. She was glad, she said, to have taken us in, because now she would have three extra pairs of hands.

The cows came as a shock. They were much bigger than they looked in pictures I had seen, and stronger too, as they jostled with each other. I imagined how easy it would be to be crushed between the heaving flanks of these creatures, or trampled beneath their huge hooves.

Mrs Bowers must have read my thoughts. "Don't fret about their pushing and shoving. They're eager to be free of their milk, is all. They'll be like lambs after."

She showed us how to grasp the udders and set up a rhythm to get the milk flowing. It wasn't as easy as she made it look and after five minutes of me tugging and the poor cow stamping and shuddering in impatience, there was only a thin trickle of milk in the pail like a strip of pale ribbon. I began to find, though, that the less I thought about it, the smoother my movements became and the more milk appeared in the pail. Appreciative now of my efforts, the cow settled down with great grass-scented sighs.

Calm settled over the cow shed as I milked and the dawn crept into the farmyard. The air smelt fresh and clear, untainted by smoke from burning buildings. These moments of peace experienced in the milking shed were so different, I knew, from the noisy, dangerous chaos I'd left behind, that I knew that our mother had been right to send us away.

I imagined her in London, leaving the air-raid shelter where she had spent the night, and returning to see if our little house was still standing, and to hear stories from neighbours of people who had been less fortunate.

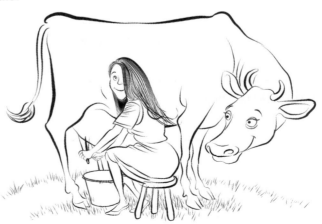

1. Who does Mrs Bowers say does all the milking? Circle your answer.

her husband she does her husband and sons

2. How many children has she taken in? Circle your answer.

1   2   3

3. Do you think the narrator had grown up in the countryside? Give a reason for your answer.

_____

4. Find and copy a word that describes how the cows move while they are waiting to be milked.

_____

5. What does the narrator imagine could happen to him in the milking shed?

_____

_____

6. What does Mrs Bowers mean when she says that the cows will be like lambs once they have been milked?

_____

_____

7–8. Find and write down two phrases which describe the way things smell.

_____

_____

9. Why do you think the child's mother has sent them away?

_____

_____

10. When do you think the story is set?

_____

_____ /10

Add the **prefix** *auto* or *bi* to these words.

11. _____graph

12. _____mobile

13. _____cycle

14. _____focal

15. _____biography

16. _____lingual

17. _____monthly

18. _____pilot

/8

Write this sentence again, adding the capital letters and **punctuation**.

19–22. landing in egypt we couldnt believe how hot it was

_____

_____

/4

Write down a short **definition** for each word.

23. precious   _____

24. eventually _____

25. consonant   _____

26. brave   _____

27. local   _____

28. library   _____

/6

Write a sentence using these **homophones**.

29. great

_____

30. grate

_____

31. waist

_____

32. waste

_____

33. weight

_____

34. wait

_____ /6

Add another word to make a **compound word**.

35. hand_____

36. rail_____

37. air_____

38. motor_____

39. wind_____

40. play_____ /6

/40

PAPER 20

In the footsteps of pharaohs

Explore the wonders of ancient Egpyt on this luxury Nile cruise-and-stay holiday.   1

The Egyptian adventure begins with seven nights aboard the five-star Nile cruise-ship Rameses III, travelling from Luxor to Aswan. Trips ashore include visits to the Valley of the Kings and Queens, Karnak and Luxor temples and a tour of the Aswan high dam. All excursions are accompanied by English and Egyptian-speaking tour guides   5
who can answer your questions about the sites visited, to ensure groups get the most from their time ashore.

Rameses III was totally refurbished earlier in the year and now offers luxurious bedroom suites with Nile views, ensuite bathrooms and separate dressing areas. The new dining facilities offer guests a choice of international cuisines prepared by award-   10
winning chefs. On deck, a plunge pool and Jacuzzis provide a chance to cool off after a morning of sightseeing on shore, with a pool-side bar providing drinks and snacks throughout the day.

Guests spend the second week of their holiday in Luxor's five-star Philae Hotel. The hotel is located in a beautiful 19th century building but offers travellers the very latest   15
in comfort. Rooms are fully air-conditioned and guests can choose from three different restaurants offering a range of hot and cold meals. The hotel has two swimming pools as well as a spa and gym. Its staff are on hand round the clock to help guests to make the most of their time in Luxor and will be happy   20
to arrange excursions to the nearby Luxor museum, the night-time sound and light shows at the temple, or a trip across the Nile to see the massive Colossi of Memnon.

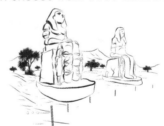

Included in the price of your holiday:

- Return flights from UK to Luxor airport
- Transfers in Egypt
- Seven nights full-board aboard Rameses III
- 11 guided excursions
- Six nights half-board at Philae Hotel
- Unlimited use of pools, spa and gym at Philae Hotel

New for this season!

An optional day trip to the Abu Simbel temples, famously moved and rebuilt during the 1960s to save them from being flooded following the construction of the Aswan Dam.

1. What do you think a *cruise-and-stay holiday* (line 1) is?

_____

_____

2. What does the word *excursion* (line 5) mean?

_____

_____

3–4. Write down two of the trips guests enjoy during the cruise.

_____

_____

_____

5. Why might it be useful for tour guides to speak both English and Egyptian?

_____

6. Why is it important for guests on a Nile cruise to be able to cool off in a plunge pool or Jacuzzi?

_____

_____

7–8. List two attractions that guests staying at the Philae hotel might want to see.

_____

_____

9. Why were the Abu Simbel temples moved in the 1960s?

_____

_____

10. Do guests at the Philae Hotel have to pay extra to use the spa?

_____

_____

/10

Complete each word with the **suffix** *al*, *ary* or ic.

11. station_____   **12.** person_____

13. atom_____   **14.** realist_____

15. diction_____   **16.** season_____

/6

Write down two words that share the
bold ending with each of these words.

17–18. prec**ious** _____   _____

19–20. spec**ial** _____   _____

21–22. **cough** _____   _____

/6

Write these sentences again, replacing one
of the repeated bold words with a **synonym**.

23. The storm was approaching **quickly** so we walked more **quickly** towards home.

_____

_____

24. The **funny** clown told us a **funny** joke.

_____

_____

25. John is **unkind** to the younger children and **unkind** to his sister.

_____

_____

26. I **cut** up an onion while Dad **cut** a pepper to go in the chilli.

_____

27. Jenny was **happy** with her present and Max was **happy** with his.

_____

_____

28. The **pretty** princess had **pretty** hair.

_____

_____ /6

Write a phrase you could use to describe each thing.

29. a sunset _____

30. a lion _____

31. a traffic jam _____

32. a waterfall _____

33. a beach _____

34. a roller coaster _____ /6

Add a suitable **adverb** to complete each sentence.

35. "Your picture is great!" said Mark, _____.

36. The stars twinkled _____ in the inky sky.

37. The boys gobbled up the chips _____.

38. I wrote the answers _____ on the test paper.

39. "Hello!" called the twins, _____.

40. James built the model ship _____ /6

/40

adjectival phrase	a group of words that describe a **noun**
adjective	a word that describes a **noun**, e.g. tiny, green
adverb	a word that describes a **verb**, e.g. kindly, prettily
alphabetical order	the order of the letters in the alphabet
antonym	a word with the opposite meaning to another word, e.g tall, short
apostrophe	a **punctuation mark** used to show possession or **contraction**
collective noun	a way of describing a group of a particular thing, e.g. flock of sheep
comma	a **punctuation mark** used to indicate a pause in a sentence, or separate items in a list
common noun	a word for an ordinary thing, e.g. book, tree
compound word	a word made up of two other words, e.g. footpath
conjunction	a word used to join parts of a sentence, e.g. and, but
consonant	the letters of the alphabet that are not **vowels**
contraction	two words joined together, where an **apostrophe** marks letters that have been removed, e.g. do not = don't
definition	the meaning of a word
diminutive	a word that describes the small version of something, e.g. piglet
exclamation mark	a **punctuation mark** used at the end of sentences to show surprise or deliver an order, e.g. Stop!
full stop	a **punctuation mark** used to send most sentences
homonym	words with the same spelling but different meanings, e.g. right handed, the right answer
homophone	a word which sounds the same but has a different spelling, e.g. maid, made
noun	a word that names a thing or person
past tense	a **verb** that describes something that has already happened
personal pronoun	a **pronoun** used to replace the names of people, e.g. she, me, him
plural	more than one of something
possessive apostrophe	an apostrophe used to indicate that something belongs to someone, or something, e.g. the girl's pen

prefix	a group of letters added to the beginning of a word to alter its meaning, e.g. re, ex, co
present tense	a **verb** that describes what is happening now
pronoun	a word that can be used in the place of a **noun** e.g. he, she
proper noun	the name of a person, place, day of the week, month of the year etc, e.g. Jill, March, Rome
punctuation	marks like **full stops**, **commas** etc. used in writing to help readers understand what they are reading
question mark	a **punctuation mark** used at the end of sentences that ask a question. e.g. Is that your coat?
root word	a word that **prefixes** or **suffixes** can be added to, to make new words
singular	just one of something
speech mark	**punctuation marks** used in pairs at the start and the end of the actual words that a character says, e.g. "It's my birthday!"
suffix	a group of letters added to the end of a word to alter its meaning, e.g. less, ful, ly
syllables	the beats in a word
synonym	a word with a similar meaning to another word, e.g. large, huge
verb	a doing or being word
vowel	the letters of the alphabet a, e, i, o and u

Progress grid

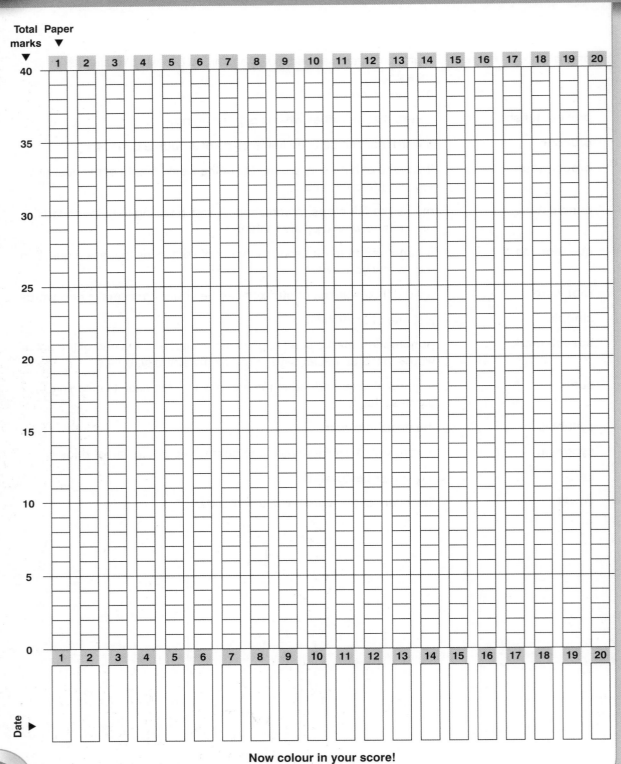

Now colour in your score!